A Consumer's Guide to
DENTISTRY

Visit our website at **www.mosby.com**

A Consumer's Guide to
DENTISTRY

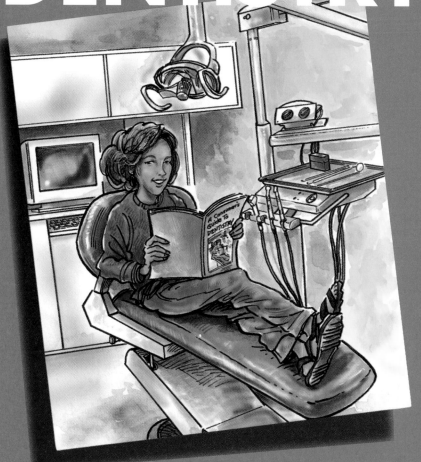

GORDON J. CHRISTENSEN, DDS, MSD, PhD, ScD

Internationally recognized Educator
Founder and Director of Practical Clinical Courses (PCC)
Co-Founder and Senior Consultant to Clinical Research Associates (CRA)
Co-Editor of CRA Newsletter
Adjunct Professor at Brigham Young University
Clinical Professor at the University of Utah
Practicing Prosthodontist in Provo, Utah

SECOND EDITION
with 508 illustrations, 469 in full color

Mosby

A Harcourt Health Sciences Company

St. Louis   London   Philadelphia   Sydney   Toronto

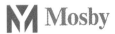

A Harcourt Health Sciences Company

Publishing Director: John Schrefer
Senior Acquisitions Editor: Penny Rudolph
Developmental Editor: Jaime Pendill
Project Manager: Patricia Tannian
Project Specialist: Anne Salmo
Book Design Manager: Gail Morey Hudson
Cover Designer: Teresa Breckwoldt

NOTICE

Pharmacology is an ever-changing field. Standard safety precautions must be followed, but as new research and clinical experience broaden our knowledge, changes in treatment and drug therapy may become necessary or appropriate. Readers are advised to check the most current product information provided by the manufacturer of each drug to be administered to verify the recommended dose, the method and duration of administration, and contraindications. It is the responsibility of the licensed prescriber, relying on experience and knowledge of the patient, to determine dosages and the best treatment for each individual patient. Neither the publisher nor the editor assumes any liability for any injury and/or damage to persons or property arising from this publication.

Mosby, Inc.
A Harcourt Health Sciences Company
11830 Westline Industrial Drive
St. Louis, Missouri 63146

Printed in the United States of America

Library of Congress Cataloging in Publication Data

Christensen, Gordon J.
    A consumer's guide to dentistry / Gordon J. Christensen.—2nd ed.
        p. ; cm.
    Includes bibliographical references and index.
    ISBN 0-323-01483-6
        1. Dentistry—Popular works. I. Title: Dentistry. II. Title.
        [DNLM: 1. Dental Care. 2. Dental Auxiliaries. 3. Dentistry. 4. Patient Education. WU
29 C554c 2001]
    RK61 .C57 2001
    617.6—dc21
                                                                                            2001030528

01 02 03 04 05 TG/RRD-W 9 8 7 6 5 4 3 2 1

Dedication

A Consumer's Guide to Dentistry is dedicated primarily to the millions of dental patients who have inadequate knowledge about dentistry to make logical decisions about the alternatives available for their oral care.

A Consumer's Guide to Dentistry is also dedicated to the hundreds of thousands of busy dentists and dental auxiliaries who do not have the time to educate patients about dentistry, but who can easily show them a few pages from this book, and then elaborate on the comments therein.

Suggestions for Dentists and Dental Auxiliary Persons

When you read the title to this book, it appears that it is intended for the buyer and user of dental services. That is correct! Although dental patients are the primary persons for whom the book is written, dentists and dental auxiliary persons must (1) place the book in locations where it will be used, (2) instruct dental staff persons about how to use it, and (3) supervise patients in its use. This book will easily pay for itself after it is used by only a few patients. *The following are some of the ways to use your* Consumer's Guide to Dentistry, *but there are many more that you can invent yourself.*

RECEPTION ROOM

One or more copies placed in your reception room provide a casual resource for your patients. Scanning through the book during a short wait for an appointment can stimulate your patients toward dental therapy or prevention about which they had no previous knowledge. Placing your name on the book will help it to remain in your office.

EDUCATIONAL AID DURING DIAGNOSTIC DATA COLLECTION

Perhaps the most significant way to use this book is during the diagnostic appointment. How many times have you stopped while educating a patient to draw a picture, search for a book, or describe verbally some technique or treatment that the patient is considering? Now you can easily find the appropriate pages in your *Consumer's Guide to Dentistry* and either let the patient read the pages alone or supervise the reading, expanding on the subjects yourself. Motivated, educated auxiliary persons can and should help in this educational process.

INFORMED CONSENT

A Consumer's Guide to Dentistry is planned to satisfy most of the needs of legal informed consent. As you have the patient read the information about the procedure that they are considering, they will also read the following related information about the procedure:

1. The treatment alternatives
2. The advantages of each alternative
3. The disadvantages of each alternative
4. The risks of the procedure they are considering
5. The relative costs of the procedure in broad descriptions on which you will need to expand because of the many fee differences among practitioners
6. The consequences of receiving no treatment at all

After your patient reads this information and sees the accompanying photographs, most informed consent questions are answered and your patient can make a more logical decision about treatment. Of course, you will have additional information that you will want to present also.

IN THE DENTAL OPERATORY

In the middle of one procedure, events often occur that change the treatment plan. It's easy to have the patient turn to the pages describing the new procedure and let the book speak for itself while you answer any additional questions. In the operatory, *A Consumer's Guide to Dentistry* makes good reading for patients who have brief waiting periods.

IN YOUR PRIVATE OFFICE

While explaining procedures to patients in a consultation, other topics often arise. *A Consumer's Guide to Dentistry* is a ready resource.

FRONT DESK

Your receptionist, scheduler, insurance person, or other business personnel are often asked about procedures that they cannot explain fully. The photos and narrative in *A Consumer's Guide to Dentistry* will help them to educate patients and to increase practice activity.

EDUCATING AUXILIARY PERSONS

New auxiliary staff persons may need additional knowledge about the many procedures in dentistry. Assigning reading in *A Consumer's Guide to Dentistry* and meeting for discussions with the new staff persons thereafter will ensure that their knowledge is more complete.

EDUCATING OTHER HEALTH PRACTITIONERS

The broad scope of dentistry is not well known among some other health practitioners. Showing the alternatives for specific oral needs to such persons will assist their understanding and will allow better cooperation and mutual respect. Giving *A Consumer's Guide to Dentistry* as a gift to physicians or other practitioners with whom you work will improve their education.

ASSISTING SPOUSES OR PARENTS TO UNDERSTAND TREATMENT

A copy of *A Consumer's Guide to Dentistry* can be sent home temporarily to allow family members or others to understand the treatment possibilities and the plans that have been presented.

A Consumer's Guide to Dentistry should become a well-used resource. I know that it can assist greatly in the education of numerous types of persons in your practice.

Acknowledgments

A very special thanks and credit go to my dental associates, **Valinda Johnston, CDA; Benette Galloway, CDA; Alycia Moore,** executive secretary; **Toni Wengreen,** continuing education director; and **Emile S. Azar, DDS, MSD,** who have spent hundreds of hours assisting in the development and refinement of this book, which I wrote in more than 15 countries over several years.

Gordon J. Christensen, DDS, MSD, PhD, ScD

CONTENTS

CHAPTER 1

How to Use This Book

Finding Solutions to Your Oral Problems

1. This book is designed to help you, the consumer of dental services.
2. When using the book correctly, you can easily find the answer to nearly every question you can imagine about your oral problems.
3. This information will allow you to discuss your questions intelligently with dental professionals.
4. After reading the sections of the book related to your oral needs, and consulting with your dental professional, you should be able to make educated decisions about your oral health care.

WAYS TO FIND THE ANSWER TO YOUR QUESTION

1. Locate your question among those that follow in this chapter. Questions are divided into major logical categories. Turn to the chapter and page indicated for your question. OR
2. The Table of Contents will lead you to the major category of your question. OR
3. If you are lost, look up the subject of your question in the index (p. 207).

FIG. 1.1   **A and B,** A fixed prosthesis (bridge) improves both appearance and function.

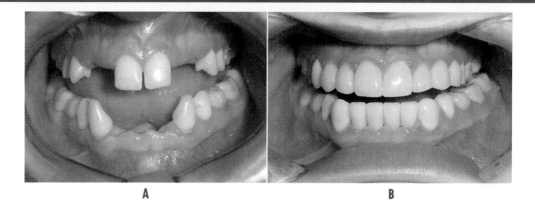

A   B

FIG. 1.2   **A and B,** Crowns (caps) on three upper front teeth have improved this person's smile.

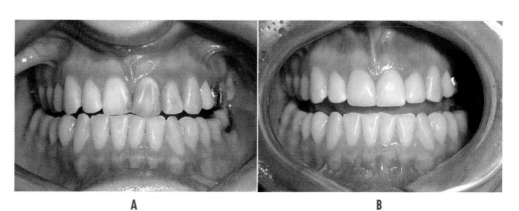

A   B

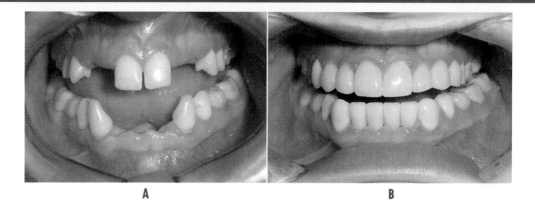

A

B

FIG. 1.3   **A and B,** Can you believe the difference four crowns (caps) make?

Question	Answer	
	Chapter	Page
Anesthetic		
Electrical Anesthesia	5	30
General Anesthetic	5	29
Hypnosis	5	30
Intravenous (IV) Sedation	5	29
Local Anesthetic	5	28
Nitrous Oxide (Laughing Gas)	5	29
Bite (Occlusion)		
Cross-bite	13	102
Teeth don't meet properly	11, 13, 14	77, 101, 119
Breath		
Foul odor from mouth	15, 16, 19	130, 133, 144
Bridges, Fixed (FIG. 1.1)		
Broken	16	145
Don't fit	16	144
Irritate gums	16	145
Large or bulky	16	144
Painful when biting	16	145
Taste foul	16	144
Wrong color	16	144

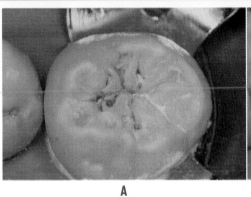

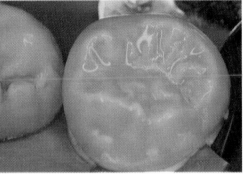

A   B

FIG. 1.4   **A and B,** The groove on the top of this tooth has been sealed, stopping future dental caries (decay).

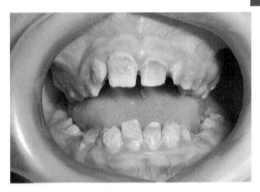

FIG. 1.5   **Occasionally, heredity factors can cause severe tooth problems; this person has amelogenesis imperfecta.**

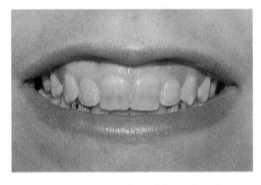

FIG. 1.6   **Drugs (tetracycline) delivered at about 1 to 2 years of age cause this unsightly tooth color in the permanent teeth.**

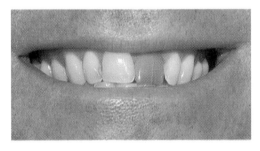

FIG. 1.7   **A dead tooth can turn dark.**

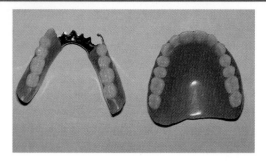

FIG. 1.8 Dentures still work, but there are better alternatives.

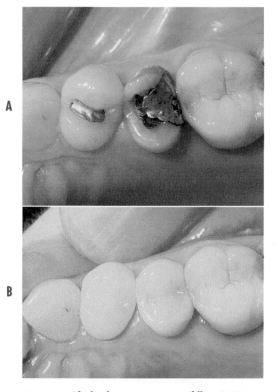

A

B

FIG. 1.9 Black silver restorations (fillings) **(A)** have been replaced with a new generation of white restorations **(B)** now available.

Question	Answer	
	Chapter	Page
Decay in Teeth		
	14, 18	113, 167
Dentist		
Finding one for your needs	3	21
Dentures, Removable (FIG. 1.8)		
Bases discolored	17	157
Bite tongue and cheeks	17	157
Broken	17	157
Can't chew with them	10, 17	63, 65, 157
Cause sore spots on gums	17	157
Clasps around teeth show too much	17	157
Food collects under them	17	156
Gums hurt when chewing	17	157
Missing teeth	17	155, 156
Pain in teeth connected to partial	17	157
Poor bite	17	157
Supporting natural teeth loose	17	157
Supporting natural teeth broken	17	157
Teeth discolored	17	157
Too tight	17	157
Face, Cheeks, Temples		
Painful	11	74
Fillings (Restorations) (FIGS. 1.9, 1.10)		
Cast gold fillings	18	172
Defective	16, 18	143, 168
Fall out	18	168
Floss catches, smells foul	18	169
Loose	18	168
Silver amalgam fillings	18	170
Taste foul	18	169
Too large	16	144
Tooth-colored fillings	18	174

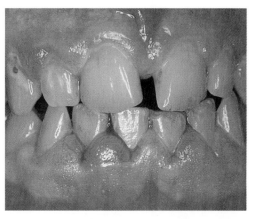

FIG. 1.10 Silver restorations still work well, but new, better-looking materials are now available.

FIG. 1.11 This woman has gingivitis (inflamed and swollen gums), commonly related to pregnancy.

How to Use This Book

Question	Answer	
	Chapter	**Page**
Gums (Gingiva) (FIGS. 1.11, 1.12)		
Bleed	12, 15	84, 129
Cover teeth	15	133
Display too much gum	8, 13	48, 104
Drainage from pimple on gums	7	37
Foul odor	15	130
Painful	15	133
Pimple on gums	7, 12	37, 86
Pus comes from gums	7, 12, 15	37, 86, 130
Receded	9, 15	58, 131
Red, magenta	15	130
Sore spots from dentures	17	157
Headaches		
	11	74
Implants		
	10	
Jaw Joints		
Clicking	11	75
Grinding	11	75
Lock open	11	75
Painful	11	75
Pop	11	75
Won't open	11	75
Jaws (Upper or Lower)		
Broken	12	88
Lower jaw too far forward or backward	8, 12, 13	50, 88, 105
Not enough bone for dentures	9, 12	59, 88
Painful	11, 12	75, 89
Upper jaw too far forward or backward	8, 12, 13	50, 88, 105
Mature Patients		
	9	
Mouth (FIG. 1.13)		
Canker sores	12	90
Cold sores	12	90
Dry	12	90
Odor	15	130, 133
White spots	12	90

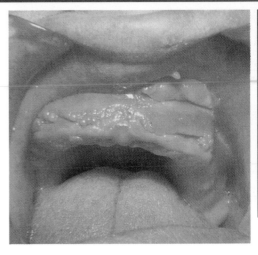

FIG. 1.12   An improperly fitting denture caused this sore mouth in a person with no teeth.

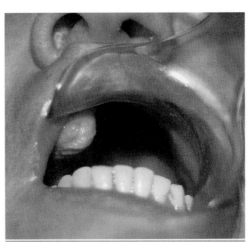

A

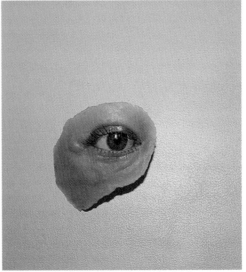

B

FIG. 1.13   This woman smoked all her life, and oral cancer developed. Her palate (A) and eye were removed. A prosthodontist (dental specialist) reconstructed her mouth and made the eye prosthesis (B), replacing part of her face also.

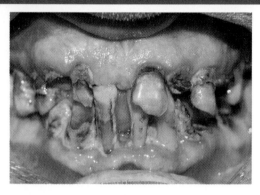

FIG. 1.14   **Every possible type of dental neglect caused this pathetic situation.**

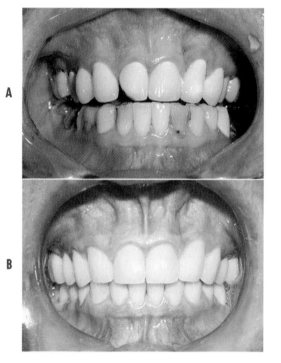

A

B

FIG. 1.15   **A** and **B,** Even the most disagreeable smile can be improved. Crowns (caps) were placed on these teeth.

A   B

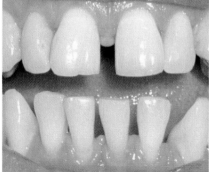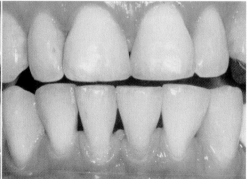

FIG. 1.16   **A** and **B,** Simple, inexpensive bonding changed this smile significantly.

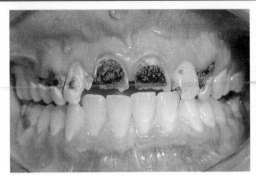

FIG. 1.17 Tooth decay (caries) is ugly, hurts, and causes teeth to be lost.

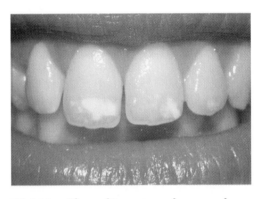

FIG. 1.18 Often, white spots can be removed easily.

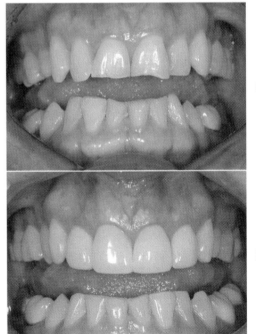

FIG. 1.19 **A** and **B,** Crooked, misshapen teeth can be greatly improved with veneers.

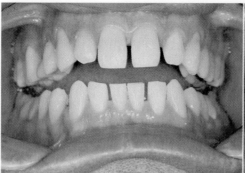
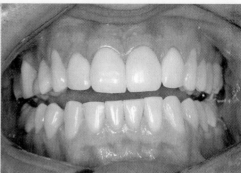

FIG. 1.20 **A and B,** Crowns (caps) on the upper teeth and simple bonding on the lower teeth greatly improve this person's appearance.

A   B

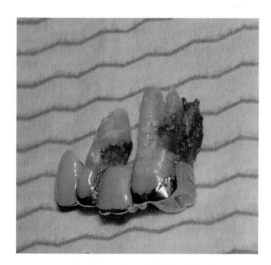

FIG. 1.21 **Fixed prosthesis (bridge) lost because of severe gum and bone disease. Note tartar on root surface.**

CHAPTER 2

Divisions in Dentistry
Types of Dentists

Many people believe that all dentists perform every aspect of dentistry. Although some general dentists provide most categories of oral services, most dentists refer patients to specialized dentists for specific treatment that they do not perform themselves. In this chapter you will learn about the various types of dentists and the services they provide. You will be able to identify the areas of dentistry that have specialists with extra education, and those that do not have specialists. Also, your vocabulary will increase, allowing you to better understand the subsequent chapters in this book.

GENERAL DENTISTRY

All dentists are general dentists when they graduate from dental school, but some complete general-practice residencies of 1 year or more to enhance their skills. Types of therapy offered by general dentists differ significantly based on their personal interest and abilities, but most or perhaps all typical oral needs can be well satisfied by a general dentist. These persons can usually be identified by one or more of the following degrees: D.D.S. and D.M.D. (equal degrees) in the United States, and, in some areas outside the United States, B.D.S., M.D., or M.B. Dental practice is called *practice* because that is actually what happens. As general dentists accumulate years of "practice" experiences, they become more competent in the areas in which they are most involved. Many dentists specialize in areas described in this chapter.

The various subcategories within dentistry have the same names as the dental specialties. These subcategories will be described as specialties to allow you to identify the name of the dental division in which your area of need is treated, and to prepare you to use dental terminology with your practitioner. Please remember that general dentists also practice most of the areas included in the following specialties. Currently there are seven recognized clinical specialties and two nonclinical specialties.

SPECIALTIES

1. Endodontics (see Chapter 7)
An *endodontist* completes at least 2 years of postdoctoral education specializing in endodontics. This area of dentistry includes treatment of teeth with diseased pulp tissue (FIG. 2.1). The inside of a tooth, called the dental pulp, is often referred to as the nerve. The pulp includes nerve tissue, blood vessels, connective tissue, and tooth regenerative cells.

Tooth pulp can be injured in numerous ways, such as a blow to the tooth, trauma of any type, an incorrect occlusion (bite), deep dental decay (caries), and inadvertent abusive dentistry. When a dental pulp is injured, it usually responds in only one way: pain. The toothache that occurs when a dental pulp is injured causes extreme pain that demands therapy to allow the patient to return to normal activity.

Pain relief is provided by having the general dentist or endodontist perform root canal therapy. Teeth usually contain one to four (and occasionally more) root canals (FIG. 2.2). A small hole is made through the top of the

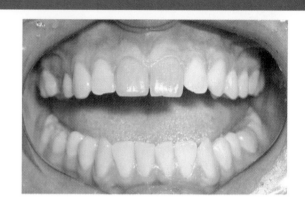

FIG. 2.1   The two upper front teeth were injured in an accident. Their pulps (nerves) have died, and thus, require root canal therapy. Usually, such teeth are discolored and require crowns (caps) later.

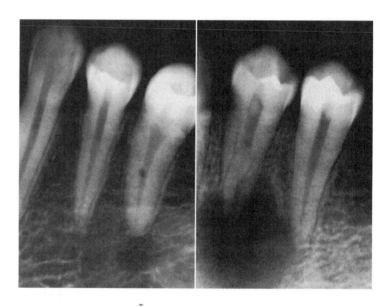

FIG. 2.2   The gray internal chambers in each tooth are root canals that house the dental pulp. (From Cohen S, Burns RC: *Pathways of the pulp,* ed 6, St Louis, 1994, Mosby.)

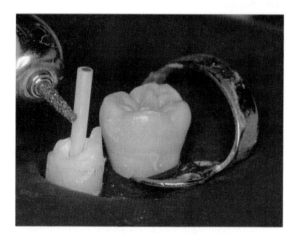

FIG. 2.3   Often, posts of various types are placed into root canal–treated teeth. These connect the weakened top part of the tooth to the root.

tooth or crown (cap) into the dental pulp, and the diseased pulp is removed. A piece of rubberlike material called gutta-percha is inserted in place of the pulp. It is cemented into the tooth with a sealant to medicate the tissue at the deepest end of the dental pulp, where it exits from the tooth into the jawbone. Other types of materials may be used to fill root canals, including various pastes and metallic or plastic reinforcements.

After the dental pulp has been removed and the remaining root canal filled, a metallic, ceramic, carbon, or fiber post **(FIG. 2.3)** may be cemented into the tooth to connect the weakened top portion (crown) of the tooth with the now hollow root.

Root canal therapy is successful in more than 95% of cases but occasionally, root canal-treated teeth are still painful. This problem is discussed in detail in Chapter 7.

Occasionally the tooth root end, deep in the bone, becomes infected in a root canal-treated tooth and requires further therapy, called an apicoectomy. In this situation a small incision is made in the gum over the root end of the tooth. Any diseased tissue is removed, and a filling is placed in the root end. The site is sutured for proper healing (see discussion of api-

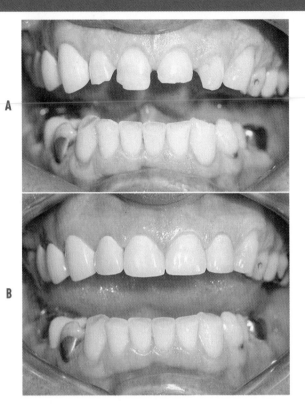

FIG. 2.4 **A** and **B,** Three of these upper front teeth required root canals, posts, and ceramic crowns (caps) after root canal therapy.

coectomy in Chapter 7, on p. 41). In addition to a post, a root canal–treated tooth may require a crown (cap) for adequate strength **(FIG. 2.4).**

2. Oral and Maxillofacial Surgery (see Chapter 12)

A person specializing in this area is an *oral surgeon* or *oral and maxillofacial surgeon.* These practitioners are dentists, or dentists with both D.D.S. and M.D. degrees, who have completed postdoctoral education in oral and maxillofacial surgery. Most of the simple oral surgical procedures **(FIG. 2.5),** including routine extraction of teeth (exodontia), are accomplished by general dentists. More complex surgery or treatment of oral-facial trauma is usually accomplished by oral surgeons. Oral and maxillofacial surgeons accomplish routine extraction of teeth; complicated extraction of teeth, including impacted (nonerupted) teeth; removal of oral tumors (growths); surgical movement of jaws to compensate for malformations, poor bite, or inadequate facial esthet-

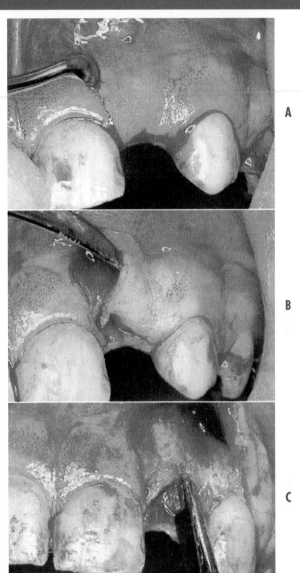

FIG. 2.5 **A to C,** Minor oral surgery such as this is accomplished by most general dentists. (From McGowan DA: *An atlas of minor oral surgery,* ed 2, London, 1999, Martin Dunitz Ltd. Copyright 1999 by DA McGowan.)

ics; and other complex oral surgery and facial plastic surgery. These specialists also treat seriously ill patients with oral surgical needs.

This field of expertise commonly overlaps with that of ear, nose, and throat (ENT) specialists and some plastic surgeons. When considering complex surgery around the face or jaws, it is advisable to consult with practitioners in all the overlapping specialty areas.

3. Oral and Maxillofacial Radiology (X-Ray)

All dentists and dental hygienists, as well as most dental assistants, have sufficient background to accomplish typical dental radiography. However, sophisticated radiographs require special expertise, such as those that show various characteristics of the skull, the temporomandibular joint, all of the teeth in one view, and many others. A few dentists limit themselves to this specialty, which requires 2 years of postdoctoral education. Numerous radiographic laboratories are staffed with well-educated technicians and/or dentists. Almost without exception these laboratories provide high-quality dental radiographic services.

4. Oral Pathology (see Chapter 12)

Oral pathologists are dentists who are involved with microscopic identification of the condition of oral tissue that has been removed surgically. These dentists, who have 2 or more years of postdoctoral education, are usually found in dental schools and hospitals. If you were to consult your dentist or dental specialist with a suspicious-looking area in your mouth, your dentist would take a biopsy (removal of a small piece of tissue, p. 91) of that area and send it to an oral pathologist for microscopic identification.

A very simple diagnostic tool is also available for superficial oral lesions. A stiff brush is rubbed over the lesion, taking some of the cells with it. This material can be observed microscopically to provide a tentative diagnosis of the suspicious lesion.

5. Orthodontics (see Chapter 13)

Many general dentists and pediatric dentists (children's dentists) perform tooth-movement procedures, but those specializing in orthodontics have completed at least 2 postdoctoral years of education in orthodontics. These practitioners are involved with prevention and treatment of malocclusion (poor bite or inadequate tooth alignment, FIG. 2.6). Most patients seeking orthodontic therapy are motivated by poor facial and tooth appearance and not by inadequate function. However, when poor tooth appearance is corrected, inadequate function is usually corrected also. Most major orthodontic cases are usually treated by or-

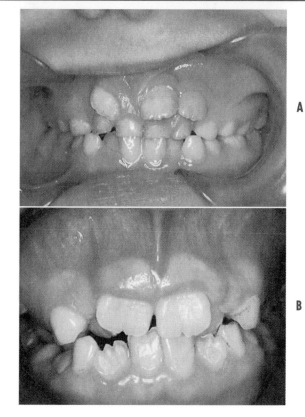

FIG. 2.6 **A and B,** These children have dentitions that are developing in malalignment and will need the services of an orthodontist. (From Tyldesley WR: *Colour atlas of orofacial disease,* ed 2, St Louis, 1991, Mosby. Copyright 1991 by WR Tyldesley.)

thodontists, but some general dentists or pediatric dentists with a special interest in orthodontics and some postdoctoral education also practice orthodontics. Regardless of the orthodontist or general dentist providing the treatment, when complex, expensive orthodontic procedures are being considered, obtaining a second opinion is suggested.

Orthodontic procedures usually require many months for completion, with multiple visits to the practitioner. Thus, you should consider the location of the practitioner relative to your home. Although many patients consider orthodontic therapy to be primarily for adolescents, many practitioners now perform adult orthodontics. Although orthodontic therapy for adults requires more time than the same treatment in the immature bone structure of adolescents, adult orthodontics is certainly possible if the patient is interested and does not mind the appearance of bands and

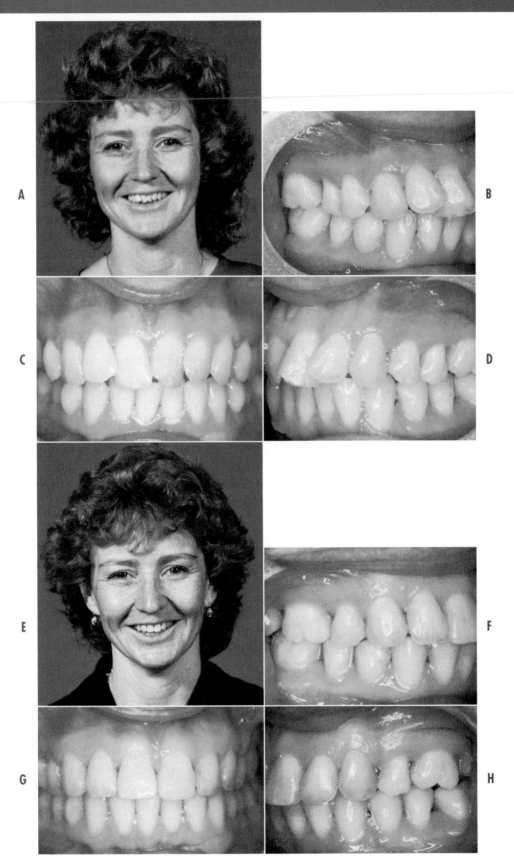

FIG. 2.7   A to H, A 27-year-old female patient is shown before and after orthodontic therapy. **Adults** *can* **have orthodontics.** (From Proffit WR and Fields HW Jr: *Contemporary orthodontics,* ed 3, St Louis, Mosby, 2000.)

Divisions in Dentistry

wires for a time while the tooth movement is taking place (**FIG. 2.7**). A new type of orthodontic therapy not requiring display of metal is now available (see p. 100) for some patients.

6. Pediatric Dentistry (see Chapter 14)

Most general dentists treat children. However, a pediatric dentist, or pedodontist, prevents or treats the special dental problems of children (**FIG. 2.8**) and has completed at least 2 years of postdoctoral education in pediatric dentistry. Although most general dentists treat routine dental problems of children, many dental conditions in children may require a specialist. An example is an infant with extreme dental caries (decay). Additionally, some children have psychological problems with dentistry. These psychological problems make routine dental treatment in a typical general dental office impossible.

When necessary, most pediatric dentists use sedation to calm children in their offices. When treating children who need general anesthetic for special physical or behavioral challenges, most pediatric dentists provide routine dental services under general anesthetic in a hospital or surgical center.

7. Periodontics (see Chapter 15)

Some general dentists treat gum and oral bone diseases, but a practitioner who specializes in this treatment is a *periodontist*—a dentist with 2 to 3 years of postdoctoral education in periodontics. These dentists treat the supporting structures of teeth (bone and soft tissue) and prevent the development of gum and bone diseases (gingivitis, periodontitis, and others).

Periodontal diseases are common in adults over 30 years of age, and because pain is not a regular symptom, patients often neglect the problem far too long. Periodontal diseases are responsible for the majority of tooth loss of adults (**FIG. 2.9**).

Periodontal diseases begin without the classic signs and symptoms of most diseases. Tartar (hard accretions) and dental plaque (a soft, whitish, creamlike substance) accumulate on tooth surfaces (**FIG. 2.10**). As this occurs, irritation of the gums is obvious because of redness and bleeding. Removal of the tartar at this time, and continued improvement of oral hygiene (plaque removal), usually causes reduced gum bleeding and redness, and a re-

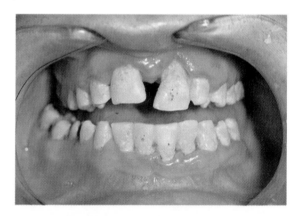

FIG. 2.9   Periodontal disease claims more adult teeth than dental caries (decay) and should be prevented.

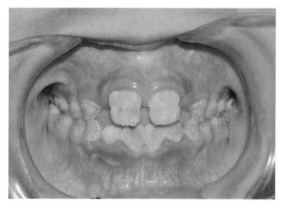

FIG. 2.8   A relatively infrequent malformation, amelogenesis imperfecta.

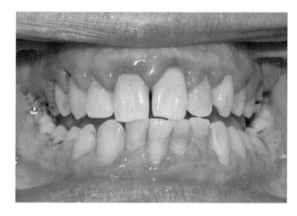

FIG. 2.10   Gross deposits, tartar, and plaque contribute to periodontal disease.

turn to healthy pink, firm gums. However, continued poor oral hygiene without professional tartar removal stimulates further gum irritation, subsequent bone loss, and eventual loss of teeth. Most periodontal diseases are preventable (see Chapter 19).

8. Prosthodontics (see Chapters 16 and 17)

Prosthodontics is the replacement of missing parts of teeth, bone, gums, or facial structures. Most general dentists perform some prosthodontic procedures, but a *prosthodontist* specializes in prosthodontics, having completed 3 or more years of postdoctoral education in one or more phases of this specialty. There are three phases of prosthodontics: (1) fixed prosthodontics (crowns and bridges) cemented onto teeth or implants in the mouth **(FIG. 2.11)**, (2) removable prosthodontics (complete or partial dentures that are removable from the mouth by the patient, **FIG. 2.12**), and (3) maxillofacial prosthetics (a less-known part of dentistry in which noses, eyes, other parts of the face, and other body parts are replaced with prostheses [artificial parts] **FIG. 2.13**). General dentists accomplish prosthodontic procedures, except for maxillofacial prosthetics. However, prosthodontists usually perform the more complex types of prosthodontic therapy.

Complex prosthodontic procedures are often necessitated by significant loss of teeth, bone, and soft tissues. Treatment plans vary widely. Also, perceived need for prosthodontic therapy varies significantly, as does expertise of dentists, prosthodontists, and laboratories that support these practitioners. It is

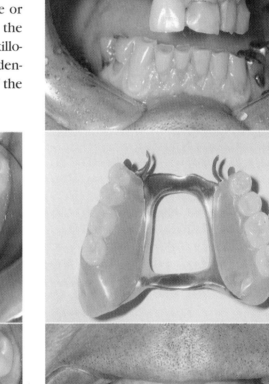

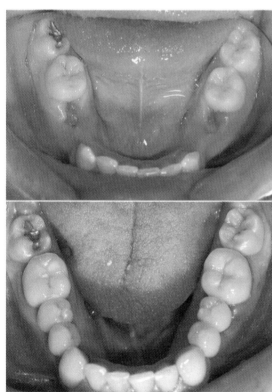

FIG. 2.11 **A and B,** Replacement of missing teeth with fixed prostheses (bridges).

FIG. 2.12 **A to C,** Crowns were placed on the upper front teeth, and a removable partial denture replaces the remainder of the upper teeth.

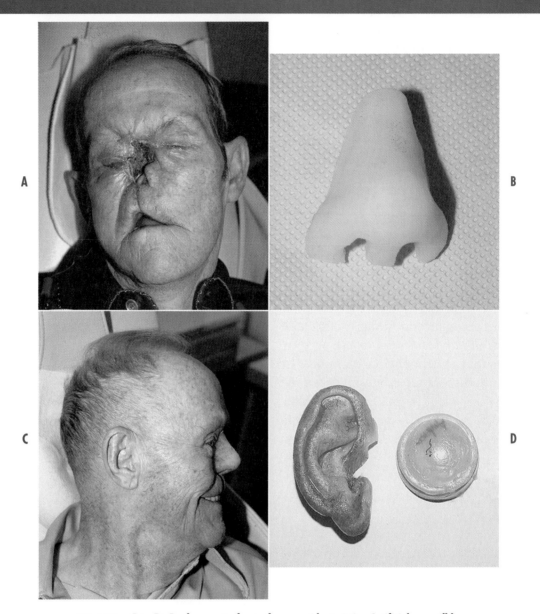

FIG. 2.13   A to D, Replacement of nose for an accident victim. Artificial ear will be held in place by metallic implants and/or glue.

suggested that multiple professional opinions be obtained before extensive prosthodontic therapy is begun.

Prosthodontic therapy usually has a predictable expected longevity directly related to quality and type of prostheses, complexity of patient need, and subsequent oral hygiene. The expected longevity should be discussed with the dentist to determine the potential cost-effectiveness of the proposed therapy.

9. Public Health Dentistry

Your geographic area has a dentist whose main goal is the most adequate prevention and treatment of dental disease for an entire geographic population. These dentists, who also have 2 or more years of postdoctoral education, usually do not practice clinical dentistry but are employed by government; they are an excellent resource for your community.

10. Nonspecialty Areas in Dentistry

The areas described above are specialties in that they have been defined as requiring additional education by various national or international organizations, such as the American Dental Association. Qualified practitioners in these areas may legally call themselves specialists, but status and education vary significantly from country to country. The

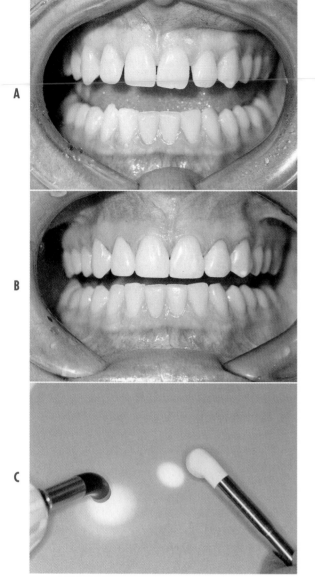

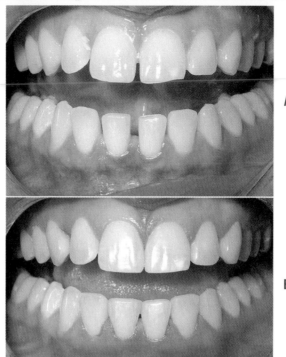

FIG. 2.15   A and B, Smiles can be greatly improved with simple, inexpensive bonding procedures.

FIG. 2.14   A to C, Cosmetic upgrading of upper front teeth requires a special curing light for the plastic placed on the teeth.

specialties previously described in this chapter are currently accepted in the United States. Check with your local dental society for differences in other countries. Other clinical areas in dentistry are identified easily, and some practitioners limit their activities to these areas. However, these subjects do not have specialty status and may not have specialty educational programs.

When you visit practitioners who indicate that their practice emphasis is limited to one of the areas described below, you must judge each situation individually based on other referring practitioners' opinions and your con-

fidence in the person involved. Addresses for organizations representing some of these areas may be found in Chapter 20, p. 188.

A. Esthetic or Cosmetic Dentistry (see Chapter 8)

Over the past 25 years many dentists have become highly interested in making their patients look as beautiful and acceptable as possible. Clinical procedures include all areas of dentistry and related health sciences, but they are usually associated with the restorative and prosthodontic areas of dentistry: bleaching teeth, bonding porcelain or resin (plastic) veneers **(FIGS. 2.14 and 2.15),** tooth-colored restorations (fillings) for posterior (back) teeth, crowns (caps), recontouring teeth, and other restorative procedures.

Various professional organizations emphasizing this part of dentistry are active internationally, and it is quite possible, but not assured, that a practitioner emphasizing esthetic or cosmetic dentistry by announcement will be more knowledgeable and/or more highly skilled than a typical general dentist in this area of dentistry.

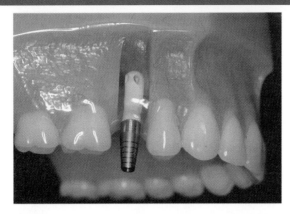

FIG. 2.16   A dental implant becomes integrated with the jawbone and can be used to support many dental reconstructive methods. In this model, the clean area around the implant shows how it fits into the bone.

B. Family Practice

This phrase is neither accepted nor denied by any organization; the designation of family practice usually infers that the general dentist is interested in serving entire families for typical routine dental needs.

C. Implantology (see Chapter 10)

Over the past 35 years, the use of dental implants (objects placed in the bone to replace teeth) has grown enormously (FIG. 2.16). Many global professional organizations exist, signifying interest and/or activity of practitioners in dental implants. Announcement by a dentist of emphasis in this area may or may not indicate special expertise in implants. There is general knowledge among dentists in any geographic area concerning fellow practitioners who have acceptable ability with implants. Implants may be used to replace one tooth, several teeth, many teeth, or all teeth. Prostheses (artificial dentures) may be (1) fixed, (2) fixed for the patient and detachable for the dentist (fixed detachable), or (3) removable.

Various national and international groups have approved implant use, and this area of dentistry is growing rapidly. If any new specialties are to be recognized officially, implantology is one of the most likely candidates.

At this time, special expertise in implants is shared by the following types of dentists (1) *surgical placement of implant:* periodontists, oral surgeons, prosthodontists, and general dentists; (2) *prosthodontic placement of prosthesis or tooth replacement over implant:* prosthodontists and general dentists. Many highly experienced general dentists or specialists accomplish both the surgical and prosthodontic aspects of dental implantology.

D. Occlusion (Dental Bite), TMD (Temporomandibular Dysfunction), and TMJ (Temporomandibular Joint) (see Chapter 11)

This area of emphasis is highly important for patients who have a problem with their occlusion (bite) or temporomandibular joints (the joint between the lower jaw and the remainder of the head). However, it is one of the most confused and confounded areas in dentistry. Numerous national and international organizations emphasize this subject, and members of one of those organizations will have more knowledge and expertise in this area than a typical general dentist.

A second opinion is always advisable in this area before therapy begins, since significant differences in professional opinion exist on almost any area of treatment.

Specialists most active in occlusion are oral surgeons, prosthodontists, and some orthodontists and periodontists.

E. Restorative Dentistry or Operative Dentistry (see Chapter 18)

Restorative or operative dentistry refers to the procedures that most patients consider the most common task of dentists restoring teeth. Why should this be an area of emphasis when every dentist learns significant depth in the subject in dental school? There are different levels of treatment in restorative or operative dentistry, and many levels of quality are observable. For example, a tooth may be restored with a typical silver filling, with an average longevity expectation of 14 years, or a well-done cast gold restoration for a lifetime (FIG. 2.17). Nearly every dentist can place a silver restoration, but only a small percentage of general dentists oriented toward operative dentistry have refined their skill to a level at

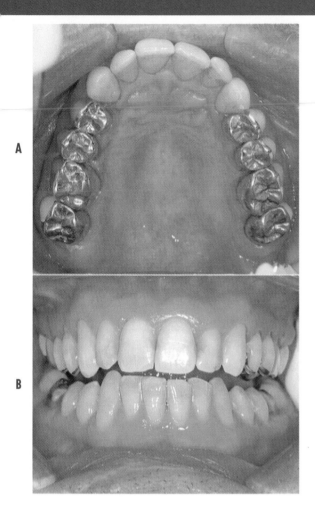

FIG. 2.17 **A** and **B,** Cast gold restorations may last for a lifetime, and they need not be unsightly when smiling.

which they are able to place a lifetime cast gold restoration.

Postdoctoral programs of 2 or more years are available in operative dentistry, and most dentists who complete these programs become dental educators. There is not a nationally recognized specialty for this area, although dentists practicing in this area are asking that their organizations be recognized as such. Chapter 3 discusses how to find excellent restorative-operative dentists.

F. Oral Medicine and Oral Diagnosis (see Chapter 12)

You may know someone who has had a strange oral disease that escaped diagnosis and proper treatment by any health practitioner. Some of these conditions are part of a systemic disease, and some are limited to the oral cavity. A few dentists limit their activity to this area; most of them are located in dental schools or hospitals.

Educational programs of 2 or more years are available in oral medicine and oral diagnosis. Most dentists who complete the programs are dental educators. Although this area is not a recognized specialty, some dentists feel that it should be, and they are lobbying for such status.

G. Preventive Dentistry (see Chapter 19)

Many dentists list preventive dentistry on their designations in some way. Many dental diseases, including the three major ones—dental caries (decay), periodontal disease (gum and bone disease), and malocclusion (bad bite or poor tooth esthetics)—can be prevented to some degree.

Although preventive dentistry is not a specialty area, it is likely that dentists designating themselves as preventive in emphasis will provide you with more information and stimulation in that area than a general dentist will.

H. Holistic Dentistry

All of medicine, including dentistry, has attempted to return to a consideration of the whole person instead of one organ, anatomical part, or disease. There has been too much emphasis on diseased parts and not on the whole person, including preventive, psychological, nutritional, and intellectual factors.

Persons calling themselves holistic practitioners are usually more interested in the whole person and will provide information and/or therapy beyond the level of your initial interest. Many are very prevention oriented. However, some practitioners have been criticized for being too involved with the fringe, less-accepted, nontraditional alternative preventions and treatments. Such judgment will be up to you, with the help of the opinions of others.

SUMMARY

Most dental patients want to find a good general dentist who has adequate knowledge about all the areas described in this chapter to be able to practice most of them and to refer you to someone else if necessary. In addition to general dentistry, you now know the names of nine recognized dental specialties (endodontics, oral and maxillofacial radiology, oral and maxillofacial surgery, orthodontics, pediatric dentistry, periodontics, prosthodontics, oral pathology, and public health dentistry) and eight other identifiable areas within dentistry. This vocabulary will help you discuss dental therapy with dental professionals. It will also help you understand the many implications involved as we discuss alternatives for dental care.

What to Consider in Your Choice of Dentists

Locating the right dentist for your needs may not be as easy as you think. As with every profession, there are those who are extremely capable and those with less experience and different interests. There are dentists whose personality characteristics would appeal to you and those who would be less acceptable.

WRONG REASONS FOR SELECTING A DENTIST

Patients often select dentists for the wrong reasons. Some of these follow.

Fees

Patients seeking low dental fees usually can find them, but the fees are usually low for a reason: often low quality or less complete service. Low-quality service can lead to irreparable situations or expensive redoing of therapy later. Similarly, high fees do not necessarily mean high quality. Don't select a dentist based on fees.

Dentist Participation in Your Company Dental Plan

Although so-called preferred providers may be competent, there is also a strong possibility that the dentists participate in the plan for various other reasons. Dentists should *not* be selected based on their participation or lack of participation in a specific dental plan.

Advertising

Some professionals advertise in various ways, including telephone books, magazines, and newspapers. Although there are some exceptions, professionals who advertise are usually no worse or better than their lower-visibility colleagues. However, patients should be cautious of professionals who advertise with unrealistic claims or strong self-aggrandizement ads. Professional advertising can be helpful, or it can be significantly misleading. Generally, most professionals still refrain from advertising.

RELIABLE WAYS TO FIND THE RIGHT PRACTITIONER

Only the health practitioner in question and a few of his or her colleagues know the competency of health services rendered by a specific person. Each practitioner has had to pass relatively difficult examinations in school, and has then had to pass rigorous national, state, or other geographic division tests. However, as in any area of endeavor, individual dentists may constantly improve themselves professionally, or they may concentrate their efforts on other areas and let their professional skills remain static. It is up to you to determine the acceptability of the practitioners you are considering, with help. I suggest that you use more than one of the following selection methods before you select a new dentist.

Dentists in Your Last Location

If you were satisfied with your previous dentist, he or she could probably help you locate a similar practitioner in your new location. Try to get at least two recommended names.

Most dentists are members of professional organizations that publish lists of member dentists in other locations. Often your previous dentist may even know someone who lives in your new location. If referrals to specific dentists are not possible, your previous dentist may refer you to a well-known, high-quality practitioner near your new area. This person can then refer you to another dentist who practices near your home. One potential negative factor: Your previous dentist may not be up to the standard you would want if you were an expert, and practitioners tend to know and associate most with professional friends who are similar to themselves.

Other Nondental Health Professionals of Your Acquaintance

Physicians, podiatrists, optometrists, veterinarians, psychologists, pharmacists, chiropractors, hospital administrators, public health officials, and others are often knowledgeable about well-respected dentists in your area. If some trusted friends in your new area are health practitioners, you might ask them if they know of dental practitioners in that area who are known for their high-quality services. Again, be careful; dentists who are prominent in civic, religious, or political groups are not necessarily the ones you want for dental care. In fact, the reverse may be the case.

Local Dental Societies

Regardless of your geographic location, dental societies represent your local group of dentists in a larger national organization. Usually these groups have a manager or an executive secretary who knows most of the dentists in your area. Look in the telephone book for the dental society; you will probably be able to reach the administrator of your local group. Although these people vary in their willingness to help a person find a dentist, many will provide a few names of their choice in your geographic area. As with any other method for locating a dentist, you must verify these suggestions with some of the other methods described in this chapter.

Dental Schools

If your city does not have a dental school, other cities close to yours might have dental schools that serve your area. If you want to find a general dentist, you might call the dental school and speak to the chairperson of operative dentistry (see Chapter 20). Ask that person to suggest a general dentist near your area. This is one of the better ways to locate a practitioner. Dental educators know the abilities of previous students or of older dentists who may be active in clinical study clubs or teaching part time at the dental school.

If you know that you need a specialist (as described in Chapter 2) you might call the chairperson of that specialty at the dental school. Excellent recommendations may be obtained in this manner.

Dental Specialists

Some of the dental specialists interact closely with general dentists and depend on the treatment delivered by those general dentists to support their specialized therapy. Such specialists usually work with many general practitioners and have in-depth personal knowledge of the abilities of specific practitioners. Staff persons in most specialist offices are pleased to recommend a few names of general practitioners close to you, and they are likely to be very good suggestions. What specialists would have the best knowledge about general dentists? Periodontists (p. 14), endodontists (p. 9), and orthodontists (p. 12) treat many patients who have received dental restorative therapy. Call the specialist's office and describe your needs; you will probably be satisfied with the suggestions offered.

Dental Laboratories

Your telephone book lists the names of dental laboratories. These firms construct the fixed prostheses (bridges), partial and complete dentures, orthodontic devices, and other laboratory work for dentists in your area. They see examples of each dentist's work, because the dentists send models to the laboratories for construction of crowns (caps), dentures, etc. The laboratory technicians become knowledgeable about the abilities of specific dentists. This referral method is especially good if you know you need fixed bridges or some form of denture. The referrals you receive from dental laboratories, based on the observations of the laboratory technicians, generally will be reliable.

Commercial Firms Recommending Health Practitioners

Many geographic areas have companies that advertise (on television and radio, in newspapers, or elsewhere) that they will recommend dentists or physicians for you. They usually have in-depth files on the practitioners, including their educational background, special practice orientations, insurance plans that they accept, and other information. Obviously, these firms must generate funds to operate. Is there a potential for conflict of interest? Of course! On the other hand, such firms will not continue to recommend dentists who have proved to be unsatisfactory for their clients. Although the companies that recommend health practitioners are one source of information about specific practitioners, you should obtain strong support from other sources before you accept their recommendations.

GET STARTED

If it has been more than 6 months since your last dental checkup, you are already late. Look over the preceding list of ways to find a dentist. Select the methods that seem to best fit your needs. Start with the simplest one and get a few names. Try another method or two and compare the names. Gradually you will gain confidence in your potential dentist, and you will be able to take that important step toward selection. All dentists are not the same, as in any other field of endeavor, but there are certainly some practitioners in your area who will satisfy your needs.

Geographic Location

Selection of a dentist solely based on geographic location is unwise. A dentist in your immediate geographic area could be perfect for you, but the reverse could be true as well. Unless you are assured by other factors that a local dentist is the right one for you, it is probably better to select a dentist because of other factors.

Personality

Many professionals appeal to patients primarily based on their gregarious, outgoing personalities. You may have met such people in civic, social, or religious situations. Although you may be able to judge your social compatibility with that of a potential dentist by such an encounter, social personality characteristics indicate almost nothing about professional skills and quality of health care services. Unfortunately, many persons select their health practitioners based on superficial social contacts. Don't! If everything else is in order, a good personality is a pleasant bonus.

Dentists of Friends

Selecting the health care professional of a friend is dangerous without other selection criteria. Too often, professionals might impress your friends while delivering treatment that would not satisfy you. However, if after you have used some of the more substantial evaluation methods described previously in this chapter to find a practitioner, having a friend who also likes and supports that practitioner is additional verification for you.

CHAPTER 4

Managed Care

Over the past several years there has been a major effort by business organizations to become involved with the administration and funding of health care. You are undoubtedly familiar with these programs as administered for your medical plans. Overall, there has been only fair to poor acceptance of the influence of these plans on the access and quality of health care. Some of these programs are now active in dentistry, but they are not nearly as dominant as they are in the other parts of medicine. This chapter provides a candid view of the various types of dental care plans that are now available in the United States as viewed through the eyes of the author, a dental practitioner, teacher, and researcher who has practiced high-quality oral care for more than 40 years. Although these opinions are those of the author, they represent the majority of opinions of the thousands of dentists to whom the author speaks each year.

Several methods of payment for dental services are available to you at this time. These major categories are described below:

FEE-FOR-SERVICE DENTISTRY

This is the type of payment for dental services many readers will remember as a child, when it was the only form of payment that was available to dental patients. You had an oral need, and you consulted with the dentist of your choice relative to that need. The dentist provided a professional opinion to you. You ac-cepted or rejected the treatment plan. The treatment was accomplished, and just as you pay for groceries or clothing, you paid for the treatment, and went home. Dental benefit plans were not available, and patients did not expect any third party to pay for their oral therapy. You selected the dentist of your choice and the quality level you could afford, and you received the treatment of your choice.

This type of oral care is still available. It is called *fee-for-service dentistry.* In fact, it is the only form of payment that many dentists will accept. In fee-for-service dentistry, you are in control of your oral health care. You select the dentist. You save the money for the service, and you pay for it. You receive the therapy of your choice that meets with your treatment preference and budget availability. However, this type of payment now constitutes only a portion of payments for oral therapy.

Some dentists who have fee-for-service practices accept so-called dental insurance funding as a part of the payment for services. However, some insurance plans will not allow the patient to receive treatment from fee-for-service dentists. In such plans, you must seek the service of so-called preferred providers who have contracts with the third-party payer.

Most high-quality dental practitioners practice fee-for-service dentistry. They cannot afford to meet the requirements for the dis-counted plans and still provide the quality level, and type of services they desire. Although there are many excellent dentists who are involved with dental insurance or dental benefit plans, you, the consumer, must be careful to analyze the potential reasons for a specific practitioner's participation in an insurance plan.

DENTAL HEALTH MAINTENANCE PROGRAMS (DHMOs)

These plans are patterned after the other medical HMO plans. A dental insurance company contracts with your employer to provide discounted oral care services for the employees of your company. The services provided by these plans are usually very minimal in nature. They provide emergency services and a few of the more rudimentary oral therapies. Almost always, they do not provide the more advanced or elective oral care services, including dental implants, veneers, orthodontics, complex crowns (caps) and bridges (prostheses) required in oral rehabilitation, major surgical services, and many other cosmetic or esthetic services. You will find that if you are involved with a dental HMO you will have some difficulty obtaining many of the services that you desire. You may find difficulty in obtaining an appointment at a time of your choice. You may find that in many offices accepting such plans the level of care you receive is different than the care you would receive from the same practitioner if you were paying a normal fee. Why do dentists become involved in DHMOs? These plans provide a specific amount of payment to the dentist for a certain time period. On many procedures, if the dentist sees the patient and provides services, he or she does not receive any additional payment. If the dentist does not see the patient, he or she receives the same amount. Is there a motivation to treat the patient? The likelihood of the patient receiving optimal dental care in a dental HMO may not be good, unless the patient has nothing to do except have an examination and go home.

It is the considered and candid opinion of the author that with very few exceptions, there is a very minimal place in a quality-oriented dental practice for DHMOs. I am pleased to report that over the past few years the number of patients involved with DHMOs has declined.

PREFERRED PROVIDER ORGANIZATIONS (PPOs)

Another type of dental plan has evolved over the past few years. In a PPO your company contracts with a dental insurance company to provide dental services for its employees for a discounted amount. The plan makes contracts with some dentists to be their "preferred providers." The discount these plans provide to you is usually about 20% off the dentist's usual fee. Some plans are more or less discounted. The plans have many limitations on the type of dental services you can receive, and usually a cap on the amount the dentist can charge. Of course the 20% discount is off the top of the maximum the dentist can charge.

A lesson in dental economics is in order. Let's say that a typical fee-for-service dentist has a fee to you for $100. You may feel that the fee is high for the time the dentist spends on your services. However, American Dental Association surveys show that the average overhead cost to run a dental office in the United States is about 70% before taxes. That leaves about 30% of the $100 for income to the dentist before taxes. Now let's discount that fee of $100 by the average PPO discount of 20%. It is now $80 coming into the dental office for your service. The dentist does not have a lower overhead in a PPO plan. In fact, there may be an even higher overhead because of the need to treat more patients to make enough money to survive at the lower income level. Therefore, there is still a $70 or more expense to serve the patient. *Take the $70 overhead off the $80 income, and you now have an astounding $10 staying with the dentist before taxes.* How do practitioners stay in practice with such a low percentage of profit? The fact is that many of them do not! They must survive on the income from their fee-for-service patients.

By cutting costs and working with more dental staff performing oral clinical services, some dentists can still provide quality services and participate in PPOs. However, in the author's opinion, the likelihood of a patient receiving consistently high-quality, complex services is not good from a dentist whose patients for the most part are involved with PPO plans.

What groups or individuals benefit from so-called dental managed care programs? You don't have to consider this question very long. Of course, the insurance companies are the major benefactors. *In the author's opinion, the patients and the dentists are the losers! Some of the plans take 20% or more of the money your company spent to provide you with services to administer the plans.* Is there a way for you to receive more of the dollars that your company designated for your dental services? YES! The following types of plans provide to you nearly all of the dollars that your company designated for you, and you actually have a choice as to what services you receive and to which dentist you may go for treatment.

INDEMNITY DENTAL INSURANCE PLANS

Because of their funding for dental services over many years, these plans are the ones responsible for the major increase in access to dental care by the American public over the past several decades. These plans have provided reasonable reimbursement for dental services, based on community-level fees. In some situations, the insurance company allows co-payment for services when it does not pay for the entire therapy, while in other plans, the dentist is allowed to charge only a given amount, and the company pays a percentage of that amount. These plans have become less attractive to dentists and patients over the past few years, since insurance companies have reduced the amount they will pay for specific services. Under close observation, such reductions have made many of the indemnity programs appear as discounted PPOs. However, with a few exceptions, indemnity insurance plans have been good.

DIRECT REIMBURSEMENT

This is one of the few types of benefit plans that actually provide advantages for both you and your dentist, and not just the insurance company!

The following example shows how direct reimbursement works. Let's say that your company wants to provide $1500 per year for your dental benefit. In a typical direct reimbursement plan, you find the dentist of your choice, and receive the services of your choice. The services need to be in line with the specifications of the plan as elected by your employer. These requirements are usually quite liberal, and not as restrictive as the previously described plans. You submit a receipt for the amount you paid to the dentist for the treatment you received. This receipt is given to a designated administrator in your company, and your company reimburses you according to the regulations of your direct reimbursement plan up to the $1500. The overhead for this type of plan is very low compared with the other plans we have discussed. It can be as low as a few percent. In direct reimbursement plans, you receive almost all of the money that was designated for your dental services!

Direct reimbursement plans have at least two disadvantages. First, you must pay the dentist and then be reimbursed by your company. This is a hardship to some patients who may not have enough cash flow to afford such an expenditure. Second, infrequently there may be an overuse of the plan by the employees that would stress your company. These disadvantages can be overcome in another type of plan described below.

DIRECT ASSIGNMENT

This type of plan is similar to direct reimbursement, with a few exceptions. Your company contracts with a local bank in your area. Your company places in the bank the amount of money it plans to spend on its dental benefit plans for a given amount of time. When you receive authorized dental therapy, your dentist submits a bill to the bank for the services. There is a small charge for the bank services, and the bill is paid to the dentist. If there is overuse of the plan by the employees for a given time period, the bank has insurance for the overage, so your company is not at risk. Direct assignment has been used successfully in Florida for several years. It overcomes the few challenges that are present with direct reimbursement.

OVERVIEW OF DENTAL BENEFITS AS DESCRIBED IN THIS CHAPTER

The information below describes the distribution of funding coming from companies to pay for dental services. This is a constantly changing area, but the trend is for fee-for-service dentistry to remain and increase slightly, dental HMOs to reduce in influence, dental PPOs to increase in influence, dental indemnity programs to decrease slightly in influence, and direct reimbursement and direct assignment to increase in influence. It is the author's preference that fee-for-service payment increase, legitimate indemnity programs increase, and direct reimbursement and direct assignment increase. Why? *These three types of payment provide the most freedom for patients to select the type of therapy they desire from the practitioner they prefer. These areas preserve the freedom of choice that has been so important in the American way of life.*

AN IDEAL DENTAL BENEFIT PLAN

The ideal plan characteristics listed in the box have been suggested by the author to third-

IDEAL DELIVERY SYSTEM*
• Patient ability to choose dentist
• All procedures included
• Patient ability to pay for extra costs over plan payment
• Simple claim forms
• Rapid payment of claims by company
• Dental society partnership in plan administration
• Dental society dominance in treatment plan review

*As proposed to dental insurance companies by Gordon J. Christensen, DDS, MSD, PhD.

party payment companies designing dental plans. Consider them and see if your benefit company provides these characteristics.

SUMMARY OF PAYMENT METHODS FOR DENTAL SERVICES

You need to determine what type of plan, if any, you have at this time.

Many employers feel obligated to provide dental services as a benefit for their employees. It appears to be logical that money designated for these plans should go to the employees, and not to dental insurance companies. Dental managed care plans (DHMOs and PPOs) take a significant amount of the money for themselves. They are in business to make a profit. When patients pay for their dental services themselves, all of the money goes for the services, and this is called fee-for-service dentistry. Direct reimbursement and direct assignment provide almost all of the money your company provides for your dental services TO YOU!

CHAPTER 5

Controlling Pain in Dentistry
Pain Control

Pain associated with the mouth has always been a subject of concern. Toothache is well known to be one of the most debilitating types of pain in the body. Because of this pain, dentists have been leaders in the development of both local and general anesthetic. Some persons believe it is necessary to feel oral pain during dental treatment. This incorrect belief has motivated many potential dental patients to avoid seeking proper periodic oral care. Is modern dentistry really that painful? What types of pain control concepts are available today? This chapter will inform you about the various methods dentists use to control pain, and it should convince you that most of *today's dentistry should be nearly painless.*

PAIN THRESHOLD

Everybody has a pain response to trauma to the body. However, the degree of pain experienced from patient to patient varies enormously. It has been estimated that about half of the population could have a simple filling (restoration) accomplished without feeling any pain. The other half cannot tolerate the slight pain associated with this restorative procedure. You probably know if you have a high tolerance to pain, or a so-called high pain threshold. If so, you are fortunate, not only because dental procedures are easier but also because many slight abuses to your body are not a problem. If you have low tolerance to pain, or a "low pain threshold," one of the following types of anesthetic is probably necessary for you to tolerate some dental procedures. Your dentist will quickly determine the level of your pain threshold, and he or she will plan your anesthesia needs accordingly.

LOCAL ANESTHETICS

Local anesthetics are the most commonly used type of pain control in dentistry (FIG. 5.1). Although you may think dentists use the old product Novocaine (Procaine), the most popular type of local anesthetic in dentistry is lidocaine hydrochloride 2%. Usually, this anesthetic has a slight amount of epinephrine (1:100,000) in it to constrict the blood vessels in the anesthetic site and prolong the duration of the anesthetic influence. This popular type of anesthetic is usually effective a few minutes after anesthetic delivery, and its duration is up to 3 hours. With very few exceptions, when this anesthetic is delivered adequately, the patient does not feel anything during treatment. Properly delivered local anesthetic should not be painful. The very small-diameter needles (FIG. 5.2), used carefully, and with preinjection topical numbing, provide simple, easy, painless anesthesia that dissipates soon after therapy is completed.

Other local anesthetic types can be selected when shorter or longer anesthesia duration is desired, or if a patient has allergies to a specific chemical type, or heart problems. Your dentist will know the best type of local anesthetic for you and will be pleased to discuss the topic

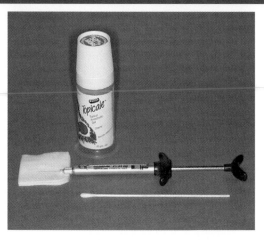

FIG. 5.1   Local anesthetic setup. Local anesthetic is highly effective, nearly painless, and has been proven for more than 100 years.

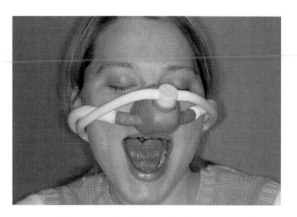

FIG. 5.3   Nitrous oxide delivery device on a patient's nose. "Laughing gas" is safe, effective, and relaxing.

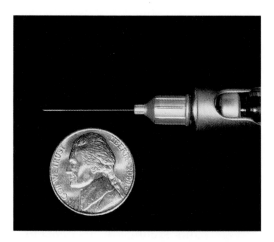

FIG. 5.2   Close-up of 30-gauge needle (by a nickel). Note the size of a modern dental needle for local anesthetic delivery. It's so small you may never feel it.

with you. There should be no reason to dread the delivery of local anesthetic.

NITROUS OXIDE (LAUGHING GAS)

About half of the dentists in the United States have nitrous oxide gas available for those persons who desire to have this relaxing chemical delivered during their oral treatment (FIG. 5.3). The nitrous oxide is monitored and delivered to you carefully. When nitrous oxide is administered properly, there is very little reason for concern. Certain groups, such as pregnant women, should avoid nitrous oxide.

INTRAVENOUS (IV) SEDATION

For some oral procedures that are potentially more painful or stressful, you can be made more comfortable by delivering a chemical into your bloodstream via a small needle inserted into a vein. Some dentists provide this service, and others do not. This procedure is not indicated for most oral needs, but your dentist can tell you if you are in need of some service for which IV sedation would be desirable.

GENERAL ANESTHETICS

Some oral procedures are best accomplished when you are asleep, under the influence of general anesthetic. Most dental procedures can be accomplished easily using local anesthetic. Probably you have had a general anesthetic before for some type of surgical procedure on your body. You know that you were required to have some dietary restrictions before the experience. Also, you were sleepy and relatively nonfunctional after the anesthesia had worn off. However, while the anesthesia was in effect, you did not feel pain.

Some dentists, especially oral and maxillofacial surgeons, deliver general anesthetic on a routine basis in their offices, a hospital, or surgical center environment. Many dentists do not use general anesthetics in their offices, and usually they will refer you to other practitioners who use general anesthetic, if you need this service.

When used properly on a healthy patient, general anesthetic is safe and totally satisfies the need for pain control during the dental procedure.

HYPNOSIS

Although hypnosis is often associated with the entertainers and a certain degree of mysticism, it is a legitimate form of pain control used in many areas of medicine, including dentistry **(FIG. 5.4)**. Only a few dentists practice hypnosis. It is estimated that about 70% of the population is capable of using hypnosis for pain control. Another 20% can be somewhat hypnotized, and 10% have personalities that do not allow successful pain control through the use of hypnosis.

Why would hypnosis be used for pain control? Many people cannot take medications because of various physical conditions or allergies. These people are in need of nonchemical anesthesia. Others have such fear of health practitioners that they cannot tolerate the delivery of anesthetics using needles. For psychological reasons these people are well treated while using hypnosis. How does hypnosis work? Usually the dentist will have a pretreatment session with the patient to introduce him or her to hypnosis and to test the patient's susceptibility to hypnotic techniques. Assuming the patient is capable of being hypnotized, the dentist will place the patient in a hypnotic trance for the oral procedure. It is amazing to see how this concept works. Under hypnosis, patients can control salivary flow, blood flow, pulse rate, and most importantly, pain. If this concept interests you, ask your dentist about availability of hypnosis for oral treatment in your community.

ELECTRICAL ANESTHESIA

This anesthesia concept is used by some dentists, and it is successful on many patients for minor oral procedures. Electrical anesthesia is a valid medical concept used in sports injuries, muscle pain, veterinary medicine, and other situations **(FIG. 5.5)**. When using electrical anesthesia, a weak, nonpainful electrical current is delivered to the specific body site, and the electrical impulses confuse the transfer of pain along nerve pathways. In studies by the author, many patients preferred electrical anesthesia to injected local anesthetic for simple procedures because the electrical anesthesia did not require a needle penetration, and when the procedure was completed there was no lingering "numb" feeling. If this concept interests you, ask your dentist about it.

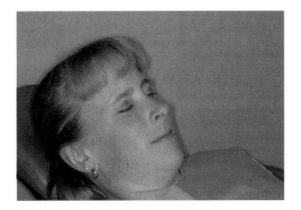

FIG. 5.4   Patient being hypnotized. If you can't have or don't want chemical anesthesia, hypnosis can work for most people. However, it requires time and patience.

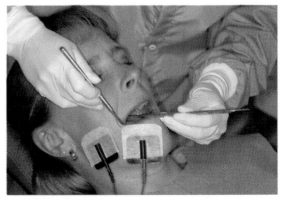

FIG. 5.5   Electrical anesthesia device placed on a patient. Electrical current, mild and painless, can confuse nerve pathways and provide an anesthetic result for some dental procedures.

SUMMARY

There are many methods to control pain during and after oral treatment procedures. If fear of pain is one of your reasons for avoiding dental therapy, perhaps this chapter has calmed your fears. Discuss your pain threshold with your dentist and decide what method of pain control would be best for you. Some dental procedures can be accomplished without any anesthetic, while others require one of the anesthesia concepts discussed in this chapter. You can be assured that an acceptable anesthesia concept is available for you to make your oral procedures as pain free as possible.

CHAPTER 6

Infection Control in the Dental Office
Infection Control

Over the past several years there has been significant controversy and lack of understanding about the possibility of contracting disease while in a dental office: Investigational reporters have produced and presented television programs that have been negative about dentists and their ability to control transmission of disease from one patient to another.

About 50 years ago, the diseases that were prevalent in the general population were different from the diseases present today. Over that time, AIDS has become a major health threat in some countries. Hepatitis B has become commonplace. Herpes has also been more prevalent. On the positive side, other diseases, such as tuberculosis, smallpox, and polio, have been greatly reduced or nearly eliminated worldwide. There are still numerous concerns among health practitioners and patients relative to the potential for transmission of disease in dental offices.

What is the current situation in most dental offices relative to infection control? Dentistry has taken on the infection control challenge with enthusiasm, backed with scientific research. The result is outstanding! Most dental offices are very safe, and you do not have to worry about contracting a disease from another patient while visiting your dentist. What has dentistry done? The following information will help you to understand the various areas of infection control now present in most dental offices. It will also provide infor-

mation for you to have a discussion with your dentist about this very important topic.

HANDPIECES

A dental handpiece is the rotary cutting instrument used by dentists to remove decay from your teeth and shape them to allow adequate restoration (FIG. 6.1). A few years ago the lay press severely criticized the dental profession, alleging that dental handpieces were not properly sterilized. The same argument could be used about dishes, knives, forks, and spoons in restaurants. Dentistry has now progressed to the point that dental handpieces are sterilized by heat before being used in your mouth. The many moving parts in handpieces break down during sterilization because of this heat. The continual replacement of dental handpieces is one of the major overhead costs your dentist incurs to provide safe treatment for you. On the positive side, sterilized dental handpieces are not a risk for you.

ENVIRONMENTAL SURFACES IN THE DENTAL OFFICE

Countertops, drawers, handles, chairs, tables, etc. collect airborne particles as well as debris from actual physical contact with contaminated materials. Similarly, such surfaces in restaurants, public restrooms, and other areas are contaminated but seldom cleaned. What has happened to these surfaces in dental

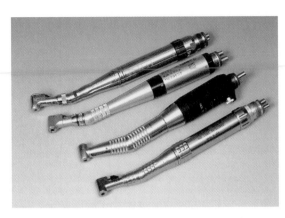

FIG. 6.1   **Handpieces. Dental handpieces are used to rotate small cutting tools that remove dental decay and shape teeth. They are sterilized using heat.**

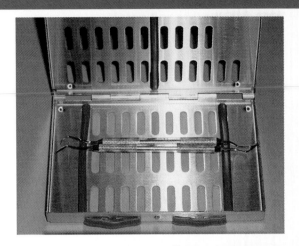

FIG. 6.3   **Instruments. Many small instruments are used in dentistry. These are sterilized by heat.**

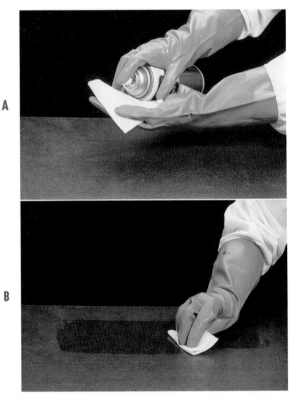

A

B

FIG. 6.2   **Environmental surfaces. A, All exposed surfaces can easily be contaminated with airborne particles. B, Wiping the surfaces with disinfectants removes this risk.**

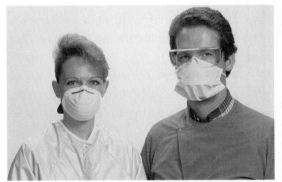

FIG. 6.4   **Face masks. Face masks prevent transfer of airborne disease from your dental therapist to you.**

offices? Employees in most dental offices wipe environmental surfaces with strong disinfectants (FIG. 6.2). It is interesting that the disinfectants that are used are available in your grocery store. Lysol sprays containing 79% alcohol are very good surface disinfectants. When the solution is sprayed into a towel and then wiped onto the surface and allowed to dry, the surface is well disinfected. Most dental offices clean environmental surfaces after the completion of each patient.

OPERATING INSTRUMENTS

Almost every dental office heat sterilizes the small instruments used in your mouth (FIG. 6.3). Sterilizers usually use heat as the sterilizing agent for dental instruments since it is efficient, effective, and relatively inexpensive. Instrument sterilization is the most adequate aspect of infection control in dental offices.

FACE MASKS

Years ago, dentists wore face masks only for surgical procedures. Over the past several decades, face masks for routine dental procedures have become very commonly used (FIG. 6.4).

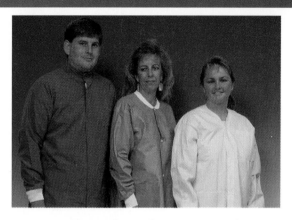

FIG. 6.5   Uniforms. Clean uniforms protect you from contaminants.

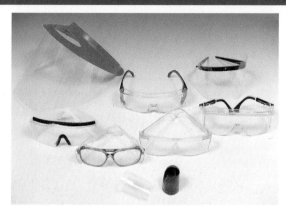

FIG. 6.6   Eye protection. There are many particles in the air when you are being treated by a dentist. Some form of eye protection is indicated, ranging from your own glasses to special glasses worn only during treatment.

What does a face mask accomplish during dental treatment? Any disease the dentist may have that is transmitted through airborne particles will be prevented by the face mask from being transmitted to you. You will be pleased to know that similarly any airborne disease you may have will be prevented from infecting the dentist. A happy additional advantage is that bad breath from the dentist is controlled also.

PROTECTIVE CLOTHING

You have probably noticed that most dentists and dental staff persons wear uniforms (FIG. 6.5). These vary from disposable uniforms that are thrown away after use, to protective uniforms that are laundered and reused. The concept of clean, protective clothing is important to you as a patient.

EYE PROTECTION

When you have oral therapy, there are millions of particles flying around the environment. Some of these particles can be especially dangerous to your eyes. Most dentists provide some form of eye protection for you (FIG. 6.6). These range from plastic covers to be used only once, to typical wide-frame safety glasses. While you are being treated, you may want to use your own glasses to avoid contaminating your eyes. Keep your eyes closed during active therapy and use eye protection.

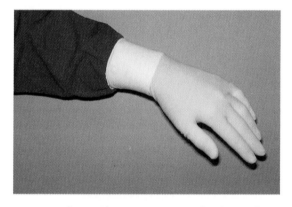

FIG. 6.7   Gloves. Gloves are now worn by almost all dentists. They are an effective disease-preventing concept.

GLOVES

If you are old enough, you will remember when dentists did not wear gloves when treating you. Such is still the case in the offices of many health practitioners other than dentists. However, in almost all dental offices, operating gloves are used routinely (FIG. 6.7). Most of these gloves are made from latex. About 90% of patients do not have any problems with latex. However, about 10% of people are allergic to latex. If you are one of those people, please inform your dentist. There are low allergenic materials used for gloves, including other forms of latex, or vinyl. What do operating gloves do for you?

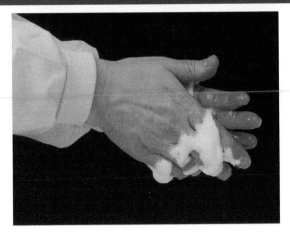

FIG. 6.8   Hand wash. Hand washes dentists use adhere to the skin and become more disinfecting as the day progresses.

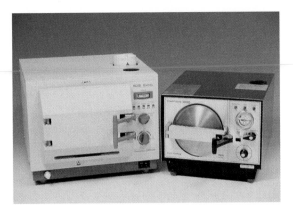

FIG. 6.9   Sterilizers. Heat sterilizers are used to kill all organisms that are contaminants on dental instruments.

Gloves are probably the most effective infection control concept, because they provide a barrier between you and the dentist. If the gloves are intact, there is very little chance for disease-producing agents to be transferred from the dentist or dental staff to you.

HAND MEDICATIONS

Most dentists and dental staff persons use a chemical named chlorhexidine gluconate as a hand wash (FIG. 6.8). This highly antimicrobiological agent combines with the skin and kills microorganisms. When the hand wash is used all day, it is cumulative, and its effect becomes more profound. When proper hand washing is combined with gloves, the chance of passing disease from the dental staff to you is negligible.

STERILIZERS

Sterilization means killing of all life. In dental offices around the world there are sterilizers of various types. Most of these use high heat in various forms for sterilization. Any items that will fit into a sterilizer are sterilized between patients (FIG. 6.9). Do the sterilizers always perform adequately? No, the sterilizers are similar to any other mechanical device. However, most dentists use sterilizer monitors

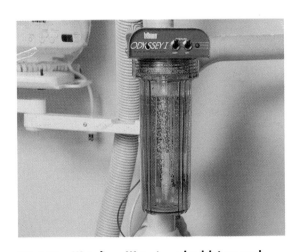

FIG. 6.10   Waterlines. Water is used to lubricate teeth while decay is removed or tooth shaping is being performed. Usually, this water is the same water that comes from your community waterlines. Dentists are beginning to place filters on these lines.

to determine if the sterilizers are working well.

DENTAL UNIT WATERLINES

You may have heard about a potential for transfer of disease from dental unit waterlines. Investigative reporters have expressed this alleged problem to the public. The organisms present in dental unit waterlines are usually increased quantities of the organisms that are present in your own community water supply. Dentists are well aware of the organisms in waterlines, and many are adding various filters to their systems (FIG. 6.10). It is highly doubtful that there is transfer of disease from one patient to another caused by dental unit waterlines or high-velocity suction systems.

SUMMARY

The possibility of contracting disease from another patient while you are in your dentist's office is highly unlikely. In fact, you are far safer going to your local dentist than eating in your favorite restaurant or using a public bathroom. Relax!

CHAPTER 7

Endodontics

Root Canals, Dead Teeth, Inside of Teeth

Each tooth has a dental pulp (FIG. 7.1), commonly called the "nerve" by patients. The anatomy of the pulp is well known to dentists. Individual teeth have divisions of the pulp called root canals. Each tooth has one to four root canals. When these small pieces of soft tissue die or become injured or infected, the resulting pain can be as debilitating as almost any other physical condition experienced by humans.

Why does a piece of diseased or dead tissue cause pain? A tooth is usually sealed externally by the outside tooth coating (enamel). Only a small opening into the supporting bone is present on the tooth end, deep within bone. When a dental pulp is diseased or dead, pulp blood flow and cellular activity increases, and there is no possibility for release of pressure from inside the tooth except into the supporting bone. The result is pain, and it is usually present when a tooth is dead or dying. However, occasionally the infection finds its way into the bone and perforates out into the soft gum tissue. The patient observes a pimplelike projection on the gums, commonly called a gum boil, and this "dead" tooth is usually not painful.

What clinical conditions are commonly observed related to dead or dying teeth?

WHAT YOU SEE OR FEEL

Conditions, Signs, or Symptoms Related to Endodontics

1. Pressure Causes Pain

(FIG. 7.2). When chewing on the suspect tooth, significant pain is experienced. Pushing on the tooth or tapping on it with a hard object creates pain. The tooth may have periods of no pain. Antibiotic therapy usually reduces or eliminates the pain for a while. Pain on pressure may be indicative of a dead or dying tooth, but it may also indicate a cracked tooth or a tooth that has had recent heavy chewing or "bruxing" on it (see Chapter 11). If your dentist finds a dead or dying tooth, you have the following alternatives:

A. Root canal (endodontic) therapy (p. 40)
B. Extraction of the tooth (p. 92)

2. Heat Causes Pain

(FIG. 7.3). If hot foods cause significant pain in a specific tooth, it usually indicates a dead or dying tooth (pulp), and you have two alternatives:

A. Root canal therapy (p. 40)
B. Extraction of the tooth (p. 92)

3. Red, Pimplelike Projection on the Gums

(FIG. 7.4). This red, pimplelike projection on the cheek side or tongue side of the tooth near the tooth root end usually indicates that the tooth pulp (nerve) is dead, and that the infection has broken through the bone to the outside. This condition creates a fistula, or canal, from the tooth root end through the gums. Often, yellow pus can be expressed from the red projection without much pain, but the pus will return until therapy is completed. Treatment for the draining fistula may include the following:

A. Endodontic therapy alone (p. 40)
B. Root canal (endodontic) therapy and an apicoectomy (root-tip amputation and root-tip filling) (p. 41) if the defect in the bone is large

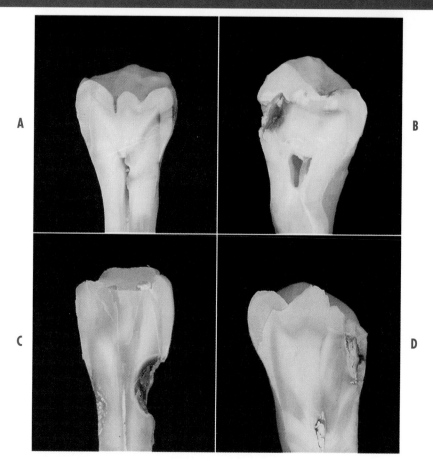

FIG. 7.1   **A** and **B** show decay on the crown portion of these extracted teeth. Decay (caries) of this size can be treated *without* root canals. **C** and **D** show decay that has progressed to the dental pulp (nerve). These teeth require root canals to be saved.

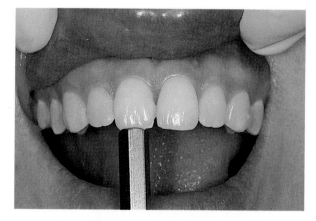

FIG. 7.2   Pushing or tapping on tooth creates pain.

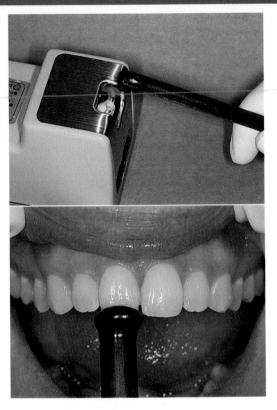

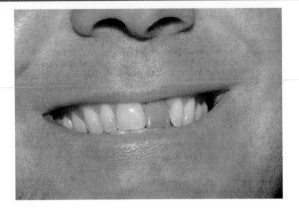

FIG. 7.5   A previously endodontically treated tooth that has turned dark.

FIG. 7.3   Heat placed on tooth to stimulate response.

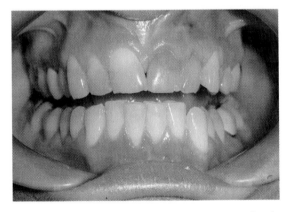

FIG. 7.4   The gray pimple on the gum is a draining fistula and requires endodontic treatment.

C. Hemisection (amputation of one or more roots) may be needed (p. 44) if the disease is especially persistent and involves only one root of a multi-rooted tooth
D. Extraction of the tooth (p. 92)

4. Tooth With a Previously Treated Root Canal Has Pain or a Draining, Pimplelike Projection

Although more than 95% of root canal treatments are successful, occasionally a few of these teeth cause subsequent pain or other problems. After discussion with your dentist, you will have several alternatives:

A. Redoing the root canal therapy (p. 40)
B. Apicoectomy (root amputation and root-tip filling) (p. 41)
C. Hemisection (amputation of one or more roots) (p. 44)
D. Extraction of the tooth (p. 92)

5. Tooth With a Previously Treated Root Canal Has Changed to a Dark Color

(FIG. 7.5). Frequently, blood or other debris are left inadvertently inside a tooth during root canal treatment. The pigments from this debris gradually cause the tooth to darken and become unacceptable in appearance. Several choices are available to patients with dark teeth subsequent to root canal therapy:

A. The tooth may be bleached by a dentist (p. 43)
B. A crown (cap) may be placed on the tooth to change the color (p. 146)
C. The tooth may be left in its darkened state (but most people do not want to have a dark-colored tooth)
D. The tooth may be removed and a prosthesis (bridge) placed (p. 149)

Endodontics

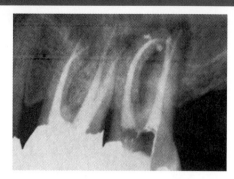

FIG. 7.6 **Endodontic therapy fills the root canal.** (From Cohen S, Burns RC: *Pathways of the pulp,* ed 5, St Louis, 1991, Mosby.)

WHAT YOUR ENDODONTIST OR GENERAL DENTIST CAN DO

Treatment Available

1. Root Canal (Endodontic) Therapy

(FIG. 7.6). When a dental pulp (nerve) is traumatized, diseased, or dead, it must be removed and replaced with a root canal filling. The filling material may vary from the most popular, rubberlike material, gutta-percha, to sterling silver, other metals, plastic, or various cements. The procedure usually requires one or two appointments. The root canal procedure typically is not painful, but some discomfort may be present during treatment and healing. In most situations the therapy is not finished after the root canal has been completed, because the tooth is now weak. Often, a reinforcing post is inserted into the tooth through the opening in the top of the tooth. Many teeth are still too weak or unpleasant looking, and a crown (cap) is required to make the tooth both functional and beautiful **(FIG. 7.7).** The minimal therapy required for a dead tooth is a root canal only. If more of the tooth is missing because of decay (caries) or old fillings, the most accepted therapy is (1) a root canal, (2) a post, and (3) a crown (cap).

A. **Advantages:** The tooth remains in your mouth, pain free. Although the cost of root canal (endodontic) therapy is significant, replacing the tooth with fixed or removable prostheses (bridges) usually costs more than the root canal therapy.

B. **Disadvantages:** There is a necessary time involvement to accomplish root canal therapy (one or more appointments): one or two additional appointments are often required to restore the dead tooth with a crown (cap). The cost is significant but well worth it.

C. **Risks:** There are not many risks to standard root canal therapy, but some exist:

1. Occasionally the tooth has more divisions of the root canals than expected, and these accessory canals are sometimes inadvertently missed by the dentist. The result is failure of the root canal therapy and continued pain requiring retreatment.

2. Infrequently, the fragile instruments used to ream or file the canals can be broken by the dentist, causing complications in achieving a successful root canal filling.

3. Occasionally, for no specific observable reason, the root canal therapy fails, requiring retreatment and/or extraction. Fortunately, this occurs less than 5% of the time.

D. **Alternative Therapy:** You do not have many alternatives. You may extract the tooth, or, in the event of a painless or infrequently painful tooth, you may postpone therapy for a short time. The tooth will not heal by itself, and root canal therapy is almost always the best selection.

E. **Cost of Various Alternatives:** Root canal therapy costs vary significantly around the world. The fee for a root canal for a single-rooted tooth costs much more than removal of the tooth. Root canal therapy costs more for a multiple-rooted than a single-rooted tooth. There is usually an additional cost if the tooth requires a post, and if a crown (cap) is needed there is a further cost. In summary, when a root canal is accomplished, that may be the only cost, but more frequently, the costs for a reinforcing internal post and a crown are necessary also.

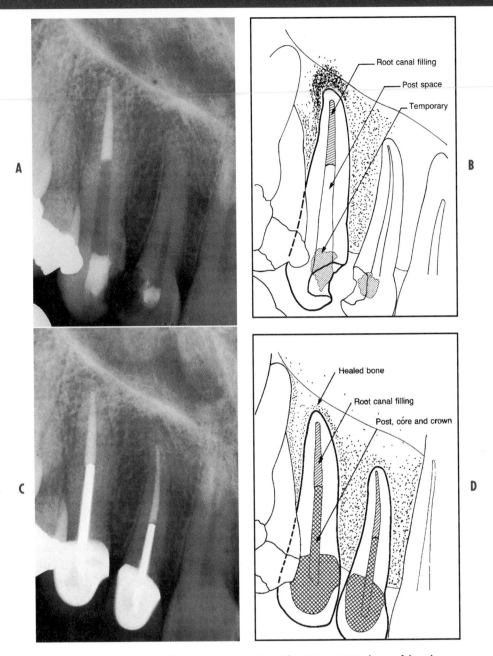

FIG. 7.7   **A to D,** Posts and crowns in teeth. (From Cohen S, Burns RC: *Pathways of the pulp,* ed 7, St Louis, 1998, Mosby.)

F. **Result of Nontreatment of a Dead Tooth:** If you do not treat a tooth with a diseased or dead pulp, continued infection will almost always occur with increased bone degeneration around the tooth, pain, and discomfort. These conditions will ultimately force you to root canal therapy or tooth extraction.

2. Apicoectomy

(FIG. 7.8). Occasionally, when viewing a radiograph (x-ray), so much disease is observable on the tooth root end that an apicoectomy is indicated **(FIG. 7.9).** A small incision is made in the soft tissue (gums) near the root end of the tooth. The diseased tissue, and usually a small amount of the tooth root end, is removed. The small opening on the root end of the

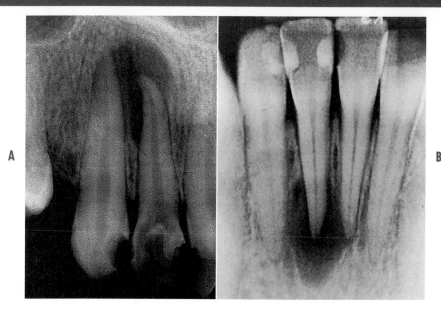

FIG. 7.8   **A and B,** Degeneration of bone around the roots of dead teeth. (From Wood NK: *Review of diagnosis, oral medicine, radiology, and treatment planning,* ed 4, St Louis, 1999, Mosby.)

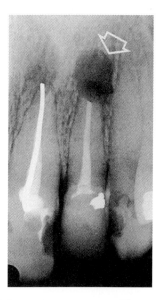

FIG. 7.9   **Apicoectomy removes a small amount of the root end.** (From Wood NK: *Review of diagnosis, oral medicine, radiology, and treatment planning,* ed 3, St Louis, 1993, Mosby.)

tooth is filled with a sealing material. The soft-tissue incision is sutured (stitched), and the sutures are allowed to remain in place for several days. Some slight to moderate discomfort is present during healing; antibiotics and medications to reduce discomfort usually are administered during the treatment and healing period.

A. **Advantages:** Surgical removal of the diseased tissue by an apicoectomy is fast, easy, and thorough, and the health status of the tooth is known immediately. Usually, healing is fast and uneventful. The tooth continues to function in your mouth.

B. **Disadvantages:** Some discomfort is involved in an apicoectomy during the healing period of a few weeks, and the cost is significant.

C. **Risks:** Apicoectomy procedures can vary from being relatively risk-free (upper and lower front teeth) to difficult and somewhat risky (some back teeth [premolars and molars]). The following risks are occasionally present: inadvertent contact with a nerve, causing a slight or total numbness in the area involved; surgical contact with the sinus cavities in the upper jaw, potentially increasing chances for sinus infection; or, infrequently, nicking or injuring teeth adjacent to the tooth being treated. Talk with your dentist about the potential risks of your apicoectomy.

D. **Alternative Therapy:** If an apicoectomy is indicated, you do not have many

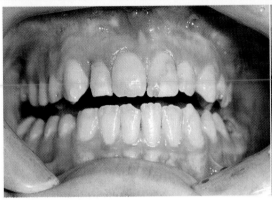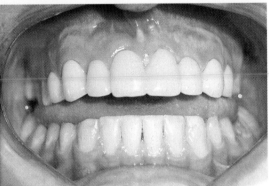

FIG. 7.10   **A and B,** Note the upper front teeth. Endodontically treated teeth that turn dark require bleaching or crowns (caps).

alternatives. You may extract the tooth, redo the root canal in the traditional manner described previously, or wait a few weeks or months to see if the tooth responds positively without treatment.

E. **Cost:** An apicoectomy is a relatively difficult procedure for the endodontist or general dentist, and the cost will be in the same range as the original root canal.

F. **Result of Nontreatment:** If a needed apicoectomy is not performed, most infected teeth will cause the surrounding bone to degenerate as a result of the presence of increased infection. However, in a small percentage of situations the infection will remain static, without increasing, over a period of weeks or months of observation.

3. Bleaching Discolored Root Canal–Treated Teeth

(FIG. 7.10). Occasionally, blue, brown, gray, orange, green, and other colors appear in teeth months to years after root canal treatment. If a crown (cap) has been placed after the root canal therapy, the color change in the tooth would make no difference. However, if a crown has not been placed, the color change in the tooth would be apparent and upsetting to the patient. Various techniques are available for bleaching discolored teeth that have had previous root canal therapy.

A. **Advantages:** Bleaching the discolored tooth is the least expensive and most conservative solution.

B. **Disadvantages:** Sometimes the discoloration reoccurs over a period of years, but it can be bleached again.

C. **Risks:** Usually there are no risks to bleaching root canal–treated teeth, but infrequently the internal tooth root degenerates, which could result in the loss of the tooth. The potential for this resorption is low.

D. **Alternatives:** The easiest, fastest alternative to bleaching is placing a crown (cap) on the tooth. The color of the surrounding teeth can be matched, and the crown will last a long time. In addition to discoloration, if the tooth has caused chronic, occasional discomfort, extraction is an alternative. Extraction requires the placement of a bridge (prosthesis) between two healthy teeth, adjacent to the missing tooth. Another alternative is leaving the tooth as is. This alternative has no significant biological or health problems; it is an appearance impediment only.

E. **Cost:** The cost of bleaching a discolored tooth is relatively low. A crown (cap) usually costs several times as much as bleaching, while tooth extraction and placement of a (prosthesis) bridge are more expensive than a crown (cap).

F. **Result of Not Bleaching the Tooth:** The only consequence is that the tooth remains unattractive in appearance.

Endodontics

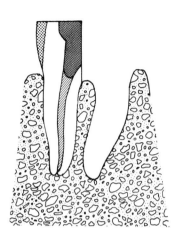
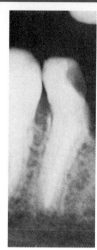

FIG. 7.11   Hemisection of tooth means removal of one or more tooth roots. (From Cohen S, Burns RC: *Pathways of the pulp*, ed 5, St Louis, 1991, Mosby.)

4. Other Less Frequently Encountered Endodontic Treatment

(FIG. 7.11). Infrequently, a multiple-rooted tooth has one or two healthy roots and one or more diseased roots. The diseased root can be removed, leaving the remainder of the tooth in place. This technique, called a hemisection, is a last attempt to save the tooth, and is usually successful. However, the cost is moderately high, and the result can be unpredictable.

SUMMARY

The major purpose of all aspects of endodontics is to retain the natural teeth. Although the cost of this therapy is relatively high, the result is a natural dentition that functions as though the teeth were completely normal. It is strongly recommended.

Esthetic Dentistry

Cosmetic Dentistry; Improving Your Smile

Most people prefer to appear "normal" in all ways, and they want their appearance to be acceptable to their friends and associates. When clothed, very few portions of the human body are observable to the public. National surveys have shown that on first meeting, the most observed portions of the body are the eyes and teeth (smile). The head and face are nearly always in view. The mouth and teeth, combined with the eyes, are the major features of facial expression. Deformed, diseased, or abnormal facial appearance can contribute to poor or misinterpreted expression and to low self-esteem. Your mouth is highly important to you, well beyond the obvious function of eating.

Modern dentistry can change and upgrade the appearance of almost any objectionable oral condition you have seen or can imagine. Practitioners from many dental specialties and subspecialties or from some of the fields associated with dentistry (such as plastic surgery) may be needed to make the changes you desire.

WHAT YOU SEE OR FEEL

Conditions, Signs, or Symptoms Related to Esthetic Dentistry

1. Discolored Teeth (Dark, Light, Spotted, Mottled, Striated)

Many conditions cause teeth to be discolored (brown, gray, orange, blue, green, white, yellow, etc.) (FIG. 8.1). Causes of discoloration include chemicals ingested during the early years of life, force or injury to the primary (baby) teeth that harm the developing permanent teeth, excess fluoride ingested during the first few years of life, drugs taken for various early-childhood diseases, metallic fillings giving color to the tooth, external stains caused by foods and drinks, and many other factors.

Persons with discolored teeth have some of the following treatment alternatives:

- A. Thorough cleaning of the teeth by a dental hygienist or dentist
- B. Bleaching (p. 51)
- C. Microabrasion (p. 53)
- D. Bonding (p. 54)
- E. Replacing metallic fillings with white restorations (fillings) (p. 173)
- F. Placing veneers (p. 55)
- G. Placing crowns (caps) (p. 146)

2. Spaces Between Teeth (Diastemas)

(FIG. 8.2). In some cultures, spaces between teeth are considered acceptable. In other cultures, spaces are not the "normal" appearance, and people want to eliminate them. These spaces are caused by teeth that are too small in relation to the size of the jaws; past removal of a tooth, causing drifting or spacing of adjacent teeth; lack of development of some teeth; orthodontic movement that did not completely close spaces; tight muscle attachments (frena) that keep teeth from coming together; and other factors.

Some spaces can be closed easily, while other spaces are more difficult to eliminate. All spaces between teeth can be eliminated if the patient sincerely desires that goal. The

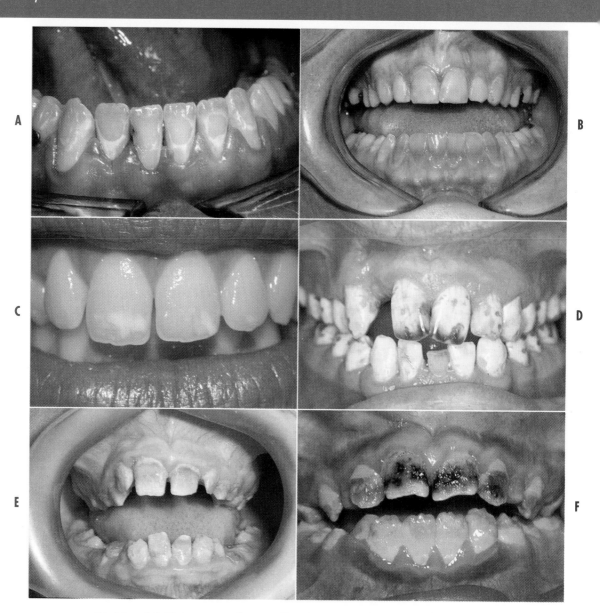

FIG. 8.1   **A-F,** Various types of genetically induced or chemically caused tooth discolorations and malformations, all of which may be improved by dentists.

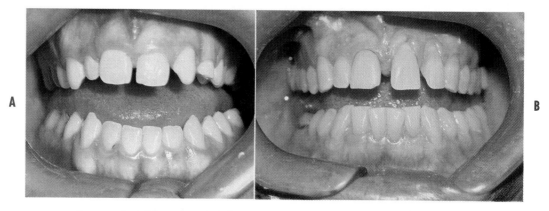

FIG. 8.2   **A** and **B,** Many people have spaces between teeth. If desired, these spaces may be closed relatively easily.

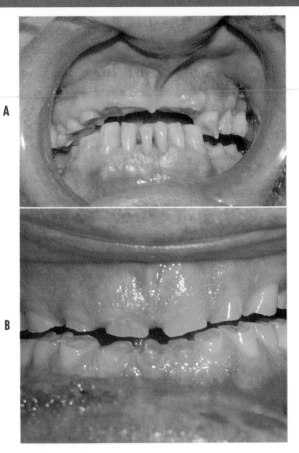

A

B

FIG. 8.3   **A and B,** Worn teeth caused by excessive grinding of teeth. Both patients can be changed to normal appearance and function.

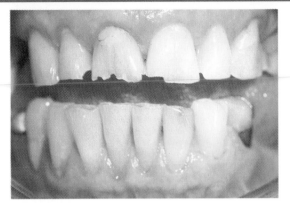

FIG. 8.4   **Broken teeth are repaired easily and relatively inexpensively.**

more common treatment alternatives for spaces between teeth include the following:

    A. Orthodontic therapy (p. 107)
    B. Bonding (p. 54)
    C. Veneers (p. 55)
    D. Crowns (caps) (p. 146)

3. Worn Teeth

(FIG. 8.3). We all cause wear of our natural teeth throughout life. Researchers estimate that normal chewing wears natural teeth a little more than the thickness of a human hair per year. Such normal wear will not be visually evident for many years into life. However, as many as one third of the population wear their teeth significantly more than normal. These people brux or clench their teeth together, grinding them excessively. They will commonly wear their teeth many times faster than normal, rapidly deteriorating their

appearance and function. Some persons may wear their teeth so much that they appear to have no teeth at all when they smile.

Persons with worn teeth often present difficult treatment challenges. One or more of the following treatment alternatives are possible:

    A. Bonding (p. 54)
    B. Placing veneers (p. 55)
    C. Placing crowns (caps) (p. 146)
    D. Orthodontics (p. 107)
    E. Periodontal surgery (gingivectomy) to remove some gum tissue, thereby making the teeth appear longer (p. 135)
    F. Placing a plastic mouth guard to reduce further tooth wear (p. 79)

4. Fractured Teeth

(FIG. 8.4). In some countries, as many as one out of two children break a front tooth during childhood. This situation is usually very upsetting to parents and can impair the child's appearance. Also, tooth fractures are not uncommon in adults. If the tooth fracture is into the dental pulp (nerve), root canal therapy (p. 40) is usually necessary before one of the treatments described below is accomplished. If the tooth fracture is below the gum, contouring of the gum tissue by gingivectomy (p. 135) may be necessary before upgrading the appearance. Only a few teeth are fractured to the degree that they must be removed, which creates a space that will need to be restored (p. 140).

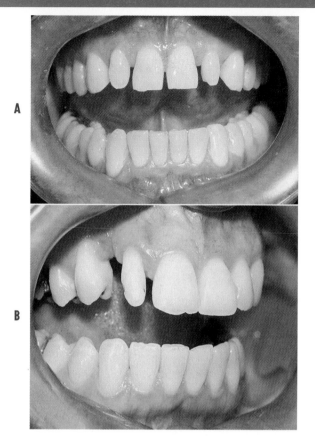

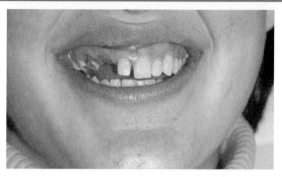

FIG. 8.6   A gummy smile can be improved.

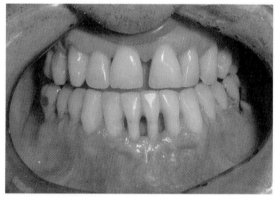

FIG. 8.5   A and B, These irregularly shaped teeth can easily be altered to normal shape.

FIG. 8.7   The lower teeth show root surfaces; correction can range from simple to complex.

One or more of the following treatment alternatives are possible for a fractured tooth:

    A. Bonding (p. 54)
    B. Placing veneers (p. 55)
    C. Placing crowns (caps) (p. 146)
    D. Extraction (p. 92)
    E. Root canal (p. 40)

5. Irregularly Shaped Teeth

(FIG. 8.5). Various conditions cause irregularly shaped teeth. They include injury to the primary (baby) teeth, which could deform the underlying permanent teeth; genetic disorders; diseases of the child or prenatal diseases of the mother during tooth development; and others.

If the spacing of teeth is relatively normal, there are at least three alternatives that provide excellent esthetic improvements for irregularly shaped teeth:

    A. Bonding (p. 54)
    B. Placing veneers (p. 55)
    C. Placing crowns (caps) (p. 146)

6. Display of Too Much Gum Tissue

(FIG. 8.6). A gummy smile is not uncommon. It is usually caused by a disproportion of the facial soft tissues (gums) and underlying bone tissue. The result can be an unpleasant appearance and an unhappy person. What can be done? The following are alternatives:

    A. Periodontal surgery (gingivectomy) (p. 135)
    B. Orthodontic treatment (p. 107)
    C. Orthognathic surgery (p. 95)
    D. Plastic surgery

7. Display of Too Much Tooth Root Surface

(FIG. 8.7). As life progresses, the gum tissues recede, and more root surface is displayed during smiling. The root surfaces usually contain more brown pigments, and this difference is often unattractive. Additionally, teeth become narrower the farther they are exposed up the root, and this narrow portion is displayed after gum recession and creates unattractive

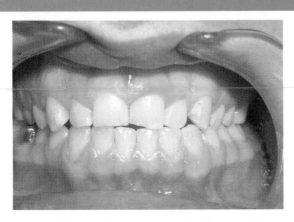

FIG. 8.8 **Short teeth present an aged smile; correction can range from simple to complex.**

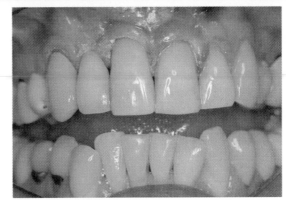

FIG. 8.9 **When teeth appear too long, there are a few alternatives for treatment.**

spaces. Such conditions are common after age 50, but fortunately they can be corrected by one or more of the following alternatives:

   A. Bonding (p. 54)
   B. Placing veneers (p. 55)
   C. Placing crowns (caps) (p. 146)

8. Display of Too Little Tooth Structure

(FIG. 8.8). Several conditions can cause excessive gum tissue that nearly grows over the teeth, making them appear too short. Sometimes the upper lip is especially long, covering the teeth nearly completely, even during smiling.

   Correction of this condition has several alternatives:

   A. Periodontal surgery (gingivectomy) to remove some gum tissue (p. 135)
   B. Bonding (p. 54)
   C. Placing veneers (p. 55)
   D. Placing crowns (caps) (p. 146)
   E. Orthognathic surgery to lengthen upper jaw (p. 95)

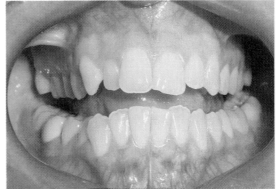

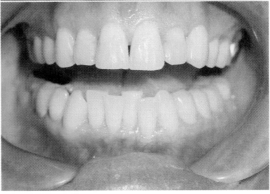

FIG. 8.10 **A and B, Irregular positioning of teeth can be corrected relatively easily.**

9. Teeth Appear Too Long

(FIG. 8.9). Sometimes teeth are especially long when they develop. Occasionally an individual's bite does not wear the teeth in a normal manner, and the teeth remain long after years of service.

   At least three alternatives are possible:

   A. Tooth recontouring (p. 54)
   B. Orthodontic treatment (p. 107)
   C. Orthognathic surgery (p. 95)

10. Teeth Not Straight

(FIG. 8.10). Many people have teeth that did not erupt in straight alignment. The major area of dentistry that deals with straightening teeth (orthodontics) is highly developed, and at least these alternatives are clear:

   A. Orthodontic treatment (p. 107)
   B. Orthodontic treatment (p. 107) and orthognathic surgery (p. 95)

Esthetic Dentistry

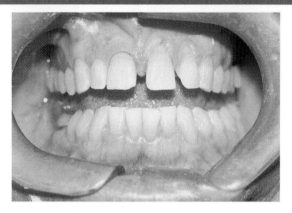

FIG. 8.11 An irregular smile creates an image that can be changed if desired.

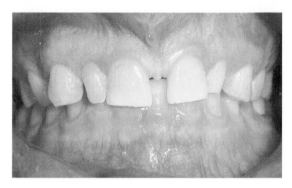

FIG. 8.12 This patient has a retruded lower jaw; this appearance can be corrected.

C. Tooth recontouring (p. 54)
D. Bonding (p. 54)
E. Placing veneers (p. 55)

11. Irregular Smile

(FIG. 8.11). Several types of smile irregularities are most common:

- The edges of the upper or lower front teeth slant uphill, making the smile line out of alignment with the face.
- The edges of the teeth are straight with the face, but the irregular gum line produces some short and some long teeth.
- The midline of the upper teeth does not coincide with the midline of the lower teeth.

The following are alternatives:
A. Tooth recontouring (p. 54)
B. Orthodontic treatment (p. 107)
C. Orthodontic treatment (p. 107) and/or orthognathic surgery (p. 95)
D. Periodontal surgery (gingivectomy) (p. 135)
E. Placing veneers (p. 55)
F. Placing crowns (caps) (p. 146)
G. Bonding (p. 54)

12. Lower or Upper Jaws Forward or Backward Compared With "Normal" Relationship

(FIG. 8.12). Such skeletal malformations occur infrequently, and they are not difficult to correct surgically. The jaws are changed in position by surgical shortening or lengthening the upper or lower jaw or both jaws. Some mi-

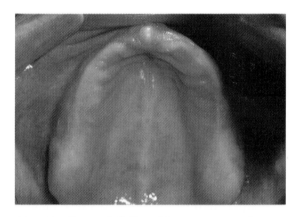

FIG. 8.13 Removal of all teeth is not common today. However, adequate artificial dentitions are available for such cases.

nor malformations may be corrected by orthodontic therapy.

The alternatives are:
A. Orthodontic treatment (p. 107)
B. Orthognathic surgery (p. 95)
C. Placing veneers (p. 55)
D. Placing crowns (caps) (p. 146)

13. Teeth Not Present

(FIG. 8.13). If all of the natural teeth have been removed, the result is highly significant both functionally and esthetically.

Current alternatives are:
A. Complete dentures (p. 163)
B. Implants followed by removable dentures (p. 66)
C. Implants followed by fixed dentures (p. 69)

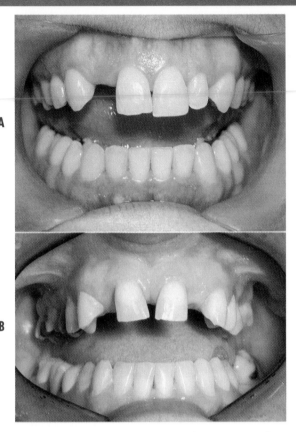

FIG. 8.14   **A** and **B,** There is no reason to have a smile impaired by missing front teeth.

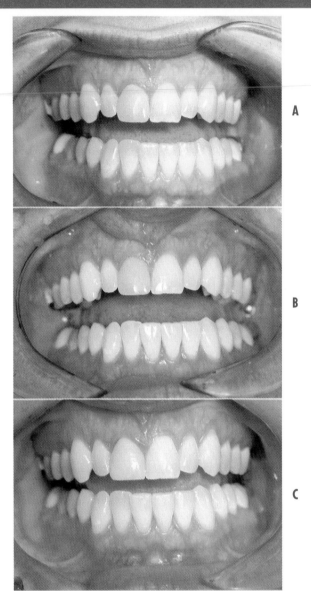

FIG. 8.15   **This patient bleached her teeth at home over 3 weeks with dentist supervision. A,** Before bleaching. **B,** After bleaching, showing one previously placed crown (cap) that did not bleach. **C,** Patient 3 years later with replacement of crown (cap) at correct new color.

14. A Few Missing Teeth

(**FIG. 8.14**). It is amazing how peculiar one appears when a few teeth are missing in a part of the mouth that is readily observable. This condition has become socially unacceptable in most developed countries. Fortunately, there are several good alternatives:

    A. Implant followed by crown (cap) (p. 72)

    B. Fixed bridge (p. 149)

    C. Bonded bridge (p. 152)

    D. Removable partial denture (p. 162)

WHAT YOUR DENTIST CAN DO

Treatment Available

Most of the procedures listed below are related primarily to improving one's appearance. They are generally considered to be esthetic or cosmetic dentistry techniques. However, some of the therapy described as treatment alternatives in the preceding section are techniques used routinely in various divisions of dentistry for reasons other than esthetic dentistry. Therefore, references listed under treatment alternatives are located in other chapters.

1. Bleaching Teeth

(**FIG. 8.15**). Some discolored teeth can be bleached well using various chemicals ap-

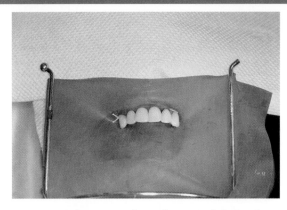

FIG. 8.16 **Whitening teeth may be accomplished in the dental office in a short time. The teeth are isolated and bleached with chemicals.**

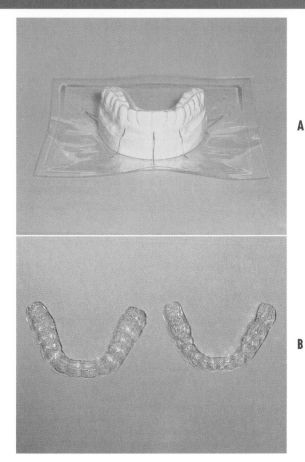

FIG. 8.17 **A and B, Custom-fitted plastic trays allow application of whitening solution to the teeth.**

plied either in the dental office or at home. When bleaching is done in the dentist's office, strong bleach is applied to the teeth to change the color of the teeth (FIG. 8.16). This technique usually requires several appointments and some time investment by the patient.

Bleaching outside the dental office has become a routine procedure (FIG. 8.17). With this type of procedure, the patient applies the bleach chemicals to the teeth using a custom-fitted, tightly adapted mouthpiece or tray that is used for 30 minutes to several hours per day for a few weeks. Although this technique requires more time, it is far more popular than the in-office bleach because it is usually less objectionable to patients than in-office procedures. Both techniques can be effective, especially when used on brown, orange, or yellow stains.

A. **Advantages:** Color change is made in the teeth without having to alter tooth structure for placement of any fillings or restorations, and the teeth remain relatively unchanged except for color. Yellow, orange, and brown stains bleach out of teeth very well. The cost of bleaching either inside or outside the dental office is relatively inexpensive compared with other methods to change tooth color.

B. **Disadvantages:** A time commitment is necessary when bleaching teeth, and some cost is involved. Some types of stains (gray, blue, striated, mottled) do not have predictable bleaching patterns and may not bleach well. However, the disadvantages of bleaching are minor compared with the advantages.

C. **Risks:** Some side effects occur occasionally when bleaching teeth. The most common ones are (1) sensitivity of teeth to cold foods or drinks for a short time after the bleaching is completed; (2) sloughing or irritation of the gums for a short time after bleaching is completed; and (3) when bleaching is done outside the dental office, the jaw joints may become sore or tired if the bleaching trays are used too much. None of these risks is serious or lasts a long time. Millions of people have undergone bleaching without significant side effects.

D. **Alternatives:** There are a few alternatives for bleaching teeth, some of which may be acceptable for your situation:
(1) Microabrasion to wear away the stains (p. 53)

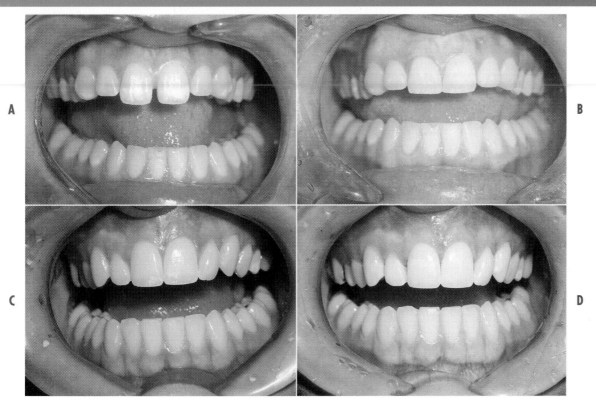

FIG. 8.18   **A and C,** White spots on upper teeth. **B and D,** Spots removed with microabrasion. Minor tooth recontouring improved the appearance also.

(2) Bonding with plastic to cover the stains (p. 54)

(3) Placing plastic or porcelain veneers over the entire front tooth surface to cover the stains (p. 55)

(4) Placing crowns (caps) to cover the stains (p. 146)

E. **Costs:** Microabrasion is a low-cost alternative. Bonding has intermediate cost. Placing veneers costs more, and crowns (caps) usually cost the most of all the alternatives.

F. **Result of Not Bleaching Teeth:** Other than continued potential for psychological damage to the person, no physiological problems are associated with leaving the teeth stained.

2. Microabrasion

(FIG. 8.18). Many tooth stains are superficial and can be treated by removing a small amount of the surface of the tooth. This microabrasion procedure is safe, not difficult, and requires a minimal amount of time. The technique adapts well to some superficial white or brown spots.

A. **Advantages:** Superficial stains may be removed rapidly, easily, painlessly, and at a relatively low cost.

B. **Disadvantages:** The technique is not acceptable for tooth discolorations that are deep within the tooth enamel.

C. **Risks:** Infrequently the treated teeth may be sensitive after the microabrasion has been finished, but this condition usually lasts only a short time.

D. **Alternatives:** Teeth with superficial stains may be treated effectively by bonding thin pieces of tooth-colored plastic over the discolorations (p. 54), or by placing veneers over the stains (p. 55). Bleaching is usually *not* an alternative to microabrasion, and crowns (caps) are typically too expensive for this need.

E. **Costs:** Bonding or placing veneers or crowns (caps) is significantly more expensive than microabrasion.

F. **Nontreatment:** Nontreatment of superficial spots on teeth has no physiological problems but may continue to

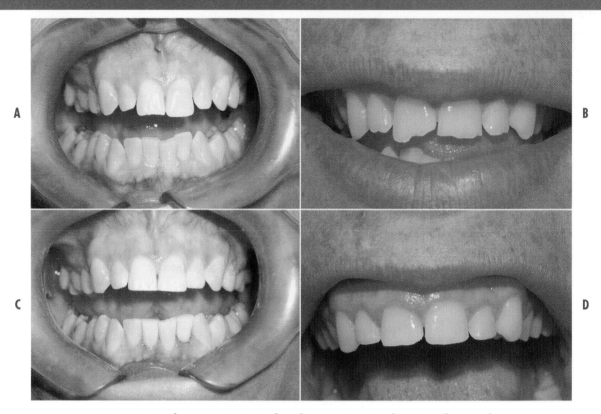

FIG. 8.19 Tooth recontouring is simple and inexpensive. **A** and **B**, Upper front teeth needing recontouring. **C** and **D**, Recontouring completed.

have a negative psychological influence on the patient.

3. Tooth Recontouring

(FIG. 8.19). The irregular appearance of teeth can often be changed to satisfy esthetic needs by slightly reshaping the teeth with abrasive instruments. This easy and inexpensive technique may be the procedure of choice for patients with only minor tooth irregularities.

   A. **Advantages:** This is a fast, simple, and inexpensive procedure that requires minimal patient commitment.

   B. **Disadvantages:** Major tooth irregularities cannot be corrected using this method.

   C. **Risks:** Patients may want to watch the dentist perform this procedure, since the slight removal of tooth contour necessary in this technique cannot be reversed. Some teeth may have minor sensitivity for a short time after recontouring.

   D. **Alternatives:** Orthodontic tooth movement is an acceptable alternative, but it takes time to complete (p. 107). Some-

times bonding (p. 54) or placement of veneers (p. 55) can also straighten teeth.

   E. **Costs:** Both bonding and placing veneers are far more expensive than tooth recontouring.

   F. **Result of Not Recontouring Teeth:** Not recontouring the teeth results in continued tooth irregularity. There are no physiological or psychological problems.

4. Bonding

(FIG. 8.20). The word *bonding* has come to mean the placement of pieces of tooth-colored plastic onto tooth surfaces to change the shape or color of teeth. The tooth enamel surfaces are etched with a mild acid so that semiliquid plastic can flow into the irregularities on the etched surfaces; the plastic will harden later. The bond of the plastic to the tooth is as strong as the bond of the tooth enamel (outside of tooth) to the tooth dentin (inside of tooth). It is a strong bond.

   A. **Advantages:** This procedure is fast (one appointment), easy, painless, and

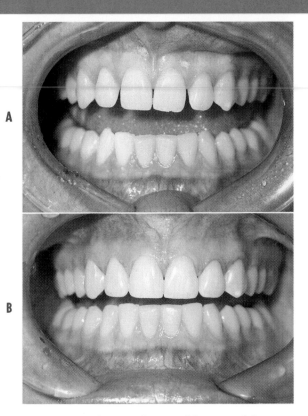

FIG. 8.20   A, The upper front teeth have unsightly spaces. **B,** A short appointment later, the spaces have been removed by bonding plastic to the tooth enamel.

relatively inexpensive; it lasts for several years. The shape and/or color of teeth can be changed in a relatively short time, influencing the patient's smile significantly.

B. **Disadvantages:** Bonded teeth need upkeep from time to time, including smoothing to remove stains and/or addition of small pieces of the bonded plastic that may have chipped away from the tooth. Eventually the bonding material must be replaced. Meticulous oral hygiene must be practiced for bonded teeth, because these teeth usually have more contour than the original teeth, and food can collect around these areas.

C. **Risks:** Chronic gum irritation and occasional dental caries (decay) around the bonding materials on the tooth occur in a few patients.

D. **Alternatives:** Placement of veneers (p. 55) is often possible to change tooth contour. Crowns (caps) can be placed (p. 146) if there is gross need for change in tooth shape or color. If only tooth color change is needed, bleaching (p. 51) or microabrasion (p. 53) are other alternatives to bonding.

E. **Costs:** Bonding is a relatively inexpensive procedure compared with placement of veneers or crowns (caps). However, bleaching and microabrasion are less expensive.

F. **Result of Not Bonding:** Forgoing bonding results in continuation of the malpositioned or discolored teeth in the mouth, and potential psychological problems. Physiological problems are usually not present.

5. Veneers

(FIG. 8.21). Veneers can significantly change the appearance of a person's smile in just two appointments. These small pieces of tooth-colored plastic or porcelain have made a significant impact in esthetic dentistry. The tooth surfaces are made microscopically irregular with a mild acid, and the laboratory-formed, correctly shaped, tooth-colored veneers are bonded onto the teeth using a tooth-colored cement. The result is usually a significant improvement in the shape and/or color of the teeth.

A. **Advantages:** Placing veneers provides major changes in teeth without cutting teeth down severely, as required for crowns (caps) (p. 146).

B. **Disadvantages:** A slight amount of tooth structure is usually removed to allow the veneer to be placed on the tooth without making the tooth too large (overcontoured). Infrequently, veneers fracture as a result of trauma, and patients are advised to use some caution when eating hard foods. Teeth with veneers require careful, thorough oral hygiene.

C. **Risks:** Because of changes in tooth contour, veneers can cause chronic gum irritation or dental caries (decay) in a few situations.

D. **Alternatives:** Depending on the situation, crowns (caps) (p. 146), bonding

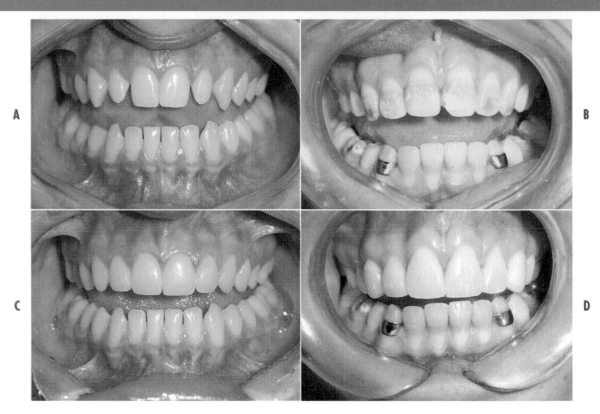

FIG. 8.21   Porcelain veneers change appearance significantly. A and B, Patients before veneers placed on the upper front teeth. C and D, Veneers on the upper six front teeth of each patient.

(p. 54), bleaching (p. 51), microabrasion (p. 53), or orthodontics (p. 107) may be accomplished instead of placing veneers.

E. **Costs:** Veneers usually cost slightly less than or the same as crowns (caps), but they are more expensive than bonding, and much more expensive than bleaching or microabrasion.

F. **Result of Not Placing Veneers:** Not placing veneers results in the continuation of the unsightly situation that existed previously. Usually, no physiological problems develop related to not placing veneers.

Other Esthetic Dentistry Treatments

Several other procedures are commonly used to make esthetic changes, but these procedures are more often associated with their specific dental specialty than with esthetic dentistry. Therefore, crowns (caps) (p. 146), orthodontics (p. 107), periodontal surgery (p. 135), and oral and maxillofacial surgery (p. 94) are discussed in other chapters of this book.

SUMMARY

The chief purpose of esthetic dentistry is to give people a more attractive facial appearance and smile, thus improving their self-esteem and confidence. This can certainly be accomplished by the procedures discussed in this and other chapters.

Oral Challenges of the Mature Person
Geriatric Dentistry

People are living longer than ever before in the history of mankind. This increased longevity has been related to excellent preventive and therapeutic medical care, public education about health, improved diet, exercise, and a reduction in smoking and alcohol consumption. Many people are living into their eighties and nineties with good health and with the ability to live their lives in a near normal manner (FIG. 9.1). But, just as 60,000 miles on your automobile tires significantly wears them, 80 years of life takes its toll on your mouth. What challenges can you expect in your oral condition as you pass into the mature years of life? This chapter describes and demonstrates numerous oral conditions of

the mature person. *You may not have all of these conditions, but you will have some of them.*

ORAL HYGIENE DIFFICULTY

The most common malady of the mature years is arthritis. How does arthritis influence oral health? A person with painful arthritic hands finds it difficult to clean his or her mouth to the meticulous level that was possible in younger years. What is the significance of inadequate oral hygiene? Dental plaque and tartar accumulations cause increased dental caries (decay) (p. 167) and periodontal disease (p. 129). If you have more difficulty cleaning your mouth than you did when you were younger, it is suggested that you ask your dentist or hygienist to suggest a mechanical toothbrush for you, and that you change your routine visits to the dentist from the standard 6-month intervals to 3-month intervals. More frequent visits will cost you more preventive dollars, but you will have less tooth and supporting structure destruction and less expense for repair (see Chapter 19).

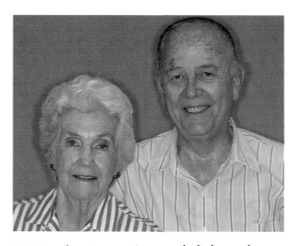

FIG. 9.1   In past generations, people died at much younger ages than they do today. With an average longevity of approximately 80 years of age, it is not uncommon to see people in their eighties who are living normal, productive, and independent lives. However, their oral problems can be challenging.

DIET

As persons move into the mature years, become more physically debilitated, and lose a few teeth, they often elect to eat softer foods. These foods are usually sticky, sugar-containing snack foods. The result of frequently eating soft, sticky, sugar-containing snack foods is a significant increase in dental caries (decay).

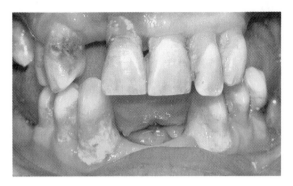

FIG. 9.2   Gums and bone have receded about ¼ inch on this patient. Note the heavy tartar and debris on the teeth. The pink color is a removable disclosing solution used to demonstrate the dental plaque accumulation to the patient. Periodontal therapy is needed, followed by replacement of missing teeth.

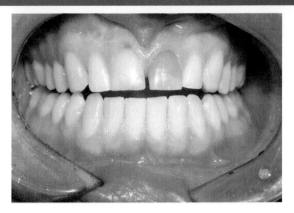

FIG. 9.3   Root canal therapy (endodontics) is needed for this patient's darkened tooth.

When such foods are consumed, they should be eaten with meals, and the mouth and teeth should be cleaned of all debris immediately after eating. This problem is especially present in nursing homes. It is suggested that when mature persons live in nursing homes, the nursing home staff persons should be instructed by the mature person's dentist on the special oral hygiene needs of their client. Currently, dental problems are one of the most significant health challenges in nursing homes, and it is related to both poor diet and inadequate oral hygiene.

GUM RECESSION (FIG. 9.2)

Gum tissues shrink (recede) as we age. This situation is unavoidable. As the gums move down the roots of the teeth, the roots are exposed. Root structure is darker in color than the enamel present on the tops of the teeth. Often, an unsightly appearance of brown-yellow roots occurs, and discriminating patients become concerned about the esthetic result. A more critical and threatening problem is root caries (decay).

TOOTH ROOT DECAY

As we move into the mature years, the gums around our teeth shrink back from the teeth,

exposing the softer, more decay-prone dentin surfaces of the teeth. This dentin is the major constituent of the tooth root. Dentin decays far faster and easier than enamel (the hard substance on the top portions of teeth). In mature persons, the combination of poor diet, gum shrinkage, and dentin exposure cause rapidly progressing, aggressive decay that often will destroy teeth within only months. Root caries (decay) is one of the most serious oral challenges facing mature adults.

ENDODONTIC THERAPY NEED

(FIG. 9.3)

Root surfaces are closer to the dental pulp (nerve) than the top surfaces of the teeth. If decay begins to destroy the root surfaces of teeth, root canal therapy can be needed within only a few months. Root canal therapy (p. 40) is expensive and destructive of tooth structure. It is to be avoided if possible by adequate oral hygiene and routine dental recare (see Chapter 19).

WEAR ON TOOTH SURFACES (FIG. 9.4)

About one third of any population has destructive habits called *bruxism* or *clenching* (p. 76). People with this condition grind their teeth, especially while sleeping. They may cause up to 100 days of wear on their teeth in only one night of grinding. Bruxism was not a

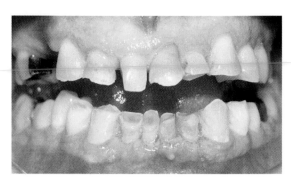

FIG. 9.4 This person has a clenching habit. He has destroyed a significant amount of tooth structure with this destructive habit. He needs major rehabilitative therapy.

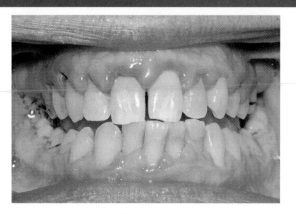

FIG. 9.6 Periodontal disease is present in most mature adults. This person has severe, ongoing periodontal disease and needs immediate treatment.

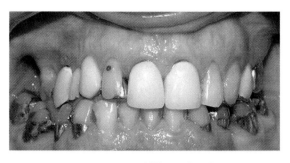

FIG. 9.5 Crowns (caps) and fillings placed many years ago have worn out in this patient. She requires major dental therapy to retain her teeth.

tooth structure and the restoration, partial clasps break, porcelain breaks from crowns (caps), and the restorative therapy degenerates. Decay starts, the bite relationship collapses, and myriad oral problems start. Mature people need to make sure they are receiving very thorough dental care even more so than they did earlier in life. Many new restorative materials containing decay-preventive chemicals are now available and they are especially indicated for mature people.

major problem when people died at age 45 or 50, but now they live beyond age 80. Often, teeth subjected to bruxism are destroyed by middle age unless occlusal bite guards are used, beginning at an early age (p. 79). If you have bruxism, you probably are well aware of this malady. Your teeth are short, worn, and potentially sensitive. If you are a bruxer, you cannot avoid tooth wear without professional help. It is imperative that this preventive, professional help be started as early in life as possible. Bruxism carried on into the mature years is catastrophic for the dentition.

OLD TOOTH RESTORATIONS (FIG. 9.5)

Restorations (fillings), crowns (caps), and other dental prostheses (partial dentures), wear out after years of service. As they wear out, openings occur between the remaining

PERIODONTAL DISEASE (FIG. 9.6)

Periodontal (gum and bone) disease (p. 129) in youth is infrequent. Periodontal disease in mature adulthood is commonplace. Mobile, spaced teeth, and foul breath often indicate that periodontal disease is present. Most mature people have some form of periodontal disease. They need professional help in the form of scaling, rinses, antibiotics, surgery, etc. They need more frequent recall appointments than they needed in their earlier years.

BONE SHRINKAGE UNDERNEATH DENTURES (FIG. 9.7)

About 40 million people in the United States have dentures. Each year the bone and gums supporting the denture shrinks. Over the period of a lifetime the bone can shrink more than half an inch, resulting in poorly adapted

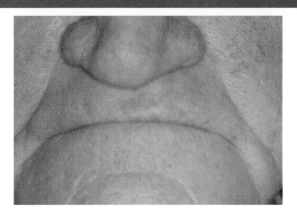

FIG. 9.7   Note the collapse of the face related to bone and gum recession under dentures. Well-made dentures can regain the facial form.

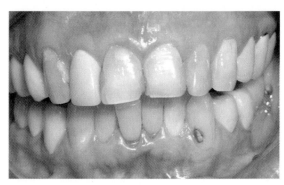

FIG. 9.8   Note the several colors of teeth and crowns (caps) in this 60-year-old person. Staining of natural teeth is present in every mature person. It can be removed with tooth-whitening techniques.

and loose dentures, poor chewing efficiency, and inadequate nutrition. Despite patients wearing the same set of dentures for decades, the average denture has a functional longevity of only about 10 years. Relines are needed every few years. For optimum health, artificial complete dentures need professional observation at least once per year and relining or remaking on a periodic basis. Your dentist can advise you concerning your own need for professional care.

DISCOLORED TEETH (FIG. 9.8)

Teeth discolor with age. This discoloration occurs because of ingestion of pigmented substances such as coffee, tea, colas, or any colored food. The color in mature teeth only has a cosmetic disadvantage, and much of it can be removed with polishing and bleaching (see Chapter 8).

SUMMARY

As with all parts of the human body, age produces a predictable degeneration of the teeth and then the supporting tissues. This chapter has discussed and demonstrated the most significant challenges that occur with your mouth in the mature years. With the help of your dentist, decide which of these challenges you face and immediately begin preventive or therapeutic care.

Implant Dentistry
Substitutes for Tooth Roots Placed into Your Jaw

Dental practitioners have tried to develop artificial teeth to be placed in the jawbones since the origin of dentistry, but in recent years activity has increased in the area of implant dentistry. Initiated by Swedish research in the 1960s, the placement of small titanium cylinders or screws into the jawbone has progressed from an experimental (and highly criticized) procedure to common usage by many dentists **(FIG. 10.1)**. The titanium-screw concept popularized implant use, but other types of implants were available much earlier. Examples are blades placed into the jawbone, with heads protruding above the gums **(FIG. 10.2)**, and subperiosteal implants placed on top of the bone, between the bone and gums **(FIG. 10.3)**. These types of implants are still used, but the screws or cylinders are more popular.

Do these tooth substitutes (dental implants) work? Yes, in the mouths of healthy people, without abusive oral habits or excessive smoking. Their ability to function rivals that of natural teeth. In severe cases they have allowed persons unable to wear conventional artificial dentures to chew well and appear normal. The most popular current concept (cylinders and screws) requires one or two clinical sessions.

1. The gum tissue is opened, and the screw-like titanium implant is placed into the

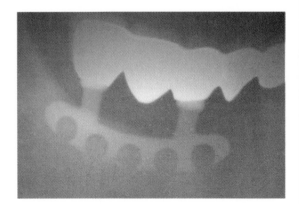

FIG. 10.2   Blade implanted in jawbone 10 years earlier.

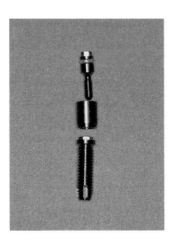

FIG. 10.1   Titanium screw-type implant goes into the jawbone, and the collar connects implant to artificial teeth held by screw.

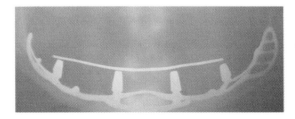

FIG. 10.3   Subperiosteal implant in lower jaw, performed 12 years earlier.

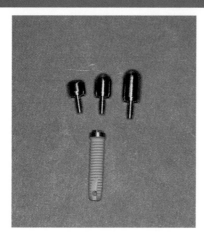

FIG. 10.4   One screw-type implant, shown with three different lengths of healing caps.

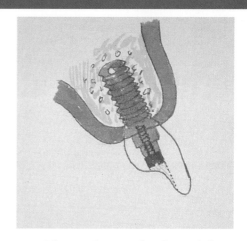

FIG. 10.6   Schematic drawing of implant and abutment head (green) and crown (cap) screwed into implant. Yellow is bone; red represents gums.

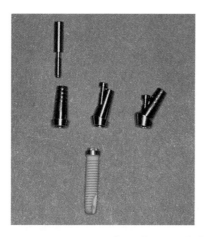

FIG. 10.5   One screw-type implant, shown with three different types of abutment heads.

bone **(FIG. 10.4)**. This implant combines with the bone as the bone cells grow into its surface. This process, which has been called *osseointegration,* takes several months. During this time, the implant is usually sealed below the gum, away from mouth fluids and debris, while it heals into place.

2. On the second appointment, a small hole is made in the gum tissue, and the implant is exposed. A healing cap is placed on the implant for a short time, and a head is placed onto the implant body **(FIG. 10.5)**. The gum tissue heals for a short time, and the dentist places some artificial teeth

(prosthesis) onto the implant(s) **(FIG. 10.6)**. These artificial teeth can be made to appear and function as well as or better than natural teeth.

On occasion, only one appointment is required. The implant is placed and allowed to protrude into the mouth. It may be restored on that appointment or at a later time.

Not all dentists provide implants. There are two distinct divisions in the implant procedure described. The placement of the implant into bone is a surgical procedure performed by oral and maxillofacial surgeons, periodontists, prosthodontists, and some general dentists. If your general dentist does not provide this service, he or she will refer you to a practitioner who performs the surgical portion of the procedure. Both portions of the implant procedure are exacting techniques requiring high skill, and experienced practitioners must be found for an optimal result. Prosthodontists or general dentists usually accomplish the second portion, or attachment of the artificial teeth (prosthesis) onto the implant(s).

If implants are so good, why doesn't everybody have them instead of natural teeth? Numerous aspects of the implant concept are complicated and difficult for dentists placing them, making the procedure less predictable than desired. Implants are expensive, and, as with natural teeth, require upkeep by patients and dentists. When implants are really needed, they do not have satisfactory substitutes. The task for you and your dentist is to determine whether your oral needs would be served best by using dental implants to replace the root structure of the natural teeth, followed by some form of prosthesis (artificial replacement) for the missing tooth structures. The following pages will help you make that decision with the help of your dentist.

WHAT YOU SEE OR FEEL

Conditions, Signs, Symptoms Related to Implant Dentistry

1. All of Your Natural Teeth Have Been Removed

(FIG. 10.7). This type of condition is called *edentulous.* Loss of all teeth is decreasing in frequency because of the use of fluoride, better diet, and improved oral hygiene. However, millions of people around the world have lost all their teeth. Unfortunately, much of this tooth loss is among those persons who are least able to afford having implants placed.

Persons without any natural teeth have several classic signs and symptoms, some of which can be helped significantly by the use of implants and tooth replacements.

A. **Collapse of Facial Form:** Edentulous persons have reduced underlying support for the muscles of the face below the nose. These muscles collapse into the void space of the mouth, giving the person an aged appearance **(FIG. 10.8).** In edentulous persons the lower jaw can close much farther than normal before it stops and hits any structures. Some edentulous persons cannot touch their upper and lower jaws together after the teeth have been removed. Few people want to have a collapsed facial appearance.

B. **Bone Shrinkage:** When teeth are removed, the bone previously holding the teeth shrinks at a fast rate, leaving only a small percentage of the supporting

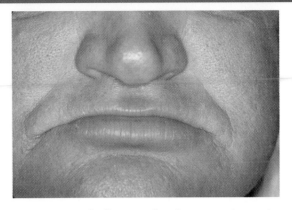

FIG. 10.7   **Facial collapse in edentulous person (no teeth present).**

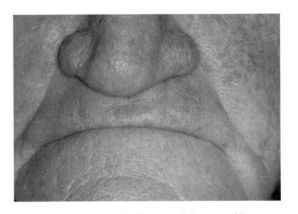

FIG. 10.8   **Severe facial collapse and thinning of lips in edentulous person. This face can be made normal again with prosthodontics (dentures).**

bone present after many years of having no teeth **(FIG. 10.9).** In the later years of life, the amount of bone remaining in the jaws may be only one third or less than that of normal bone structure. The jawbones are weak and cannot support artificial dentures well.

C. **Reduced Eating Efficiency:** Most conventional artificial removable dentures perform well for several years after tooth extraction before a significant amount of bone shrinkage has taken place. However, almost all edentulous persons eventually reach a point where the lower and sometimes upper dentures allow only a fraction of the chewing effectiveness of natural teeth. Without adequate artificial dentures,

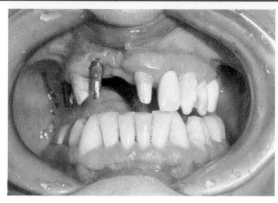

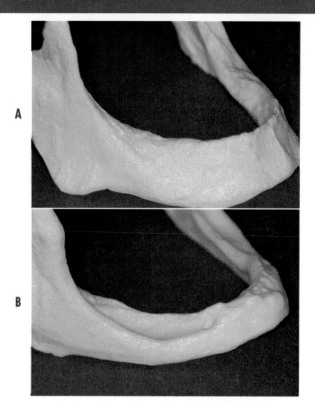

FIG. 10.10   Note enormous bone and gum shrinkage where teeth have been missing for 5 years. An implant has been placed in the area of missing teeth for a future prosthesis (bridge).

FIG. 10.9   **A,** Lower jaw after tooth removal and healing. **B,** Jaw after 15 years of shrinkage.

edentulous persons must eat only soft or liquid foods.

D. **Inability to Hold Traditional Dentures in Place:** As unavoidable bone degeneration takes place in the edentulous person, conventional dentures are difficult to keep in place in the mouth. This condition often reduces self-esteem and stimulates overall dissatisfaction with the oral part of the body.

If you are an edentulous person, you have the following alternatives:

(1) **Reline or Rebase Your Old Dentures** (p. 161). If your dentures are satisfactory except for fit, relining or rebasing your old dentures may be accomplished.

(2) **Place Conventional Complete Dentures.** Obtain conventional complete dentures without any surgical changes in your mouth (p. 163).

(3) **Change Soft Tissues in Mouth Surgically.** You may have the soft tissues in your mouth changed surgically (p. 97), providing more bone support for a new denture; then obtain new conventional dentures.

(4) **Place Implants and Construct a Removable Denture.** Place implants, allow healing, and obtain a *removable denture* that is supported and retained by the implants. You can remove this prosthesis each day for cleaning (p. 66).

(5) **Place Implants and Construct a Fixed Denture.** Place implants and construct a *fixed denture* that is supported and retained by the implants. You cannot remove this prosthesis yourself. Some of these prostheses are removable by the dentist only, and some are cemented into place and are not removable at all unless required by breakage (p. 69).

(6) **Do Nothing.** If you elect to do nothing, the signs and symptoms will continue to get worse until you are forced to do something.

2. Some of Your Natural Teeth Have Been Removed

(FIG. 10.10). A high percentage of people lose some of their natural teeth during their lifetime because of accidents, tooth decay, gum and bone disease, or other reasons. Although there are numerous solutions for replacing several teeth, dental implants are an excellent alternative.

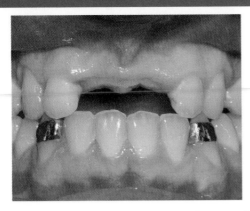

FIG. 10.11   Do you like this smile? It can be repaired.

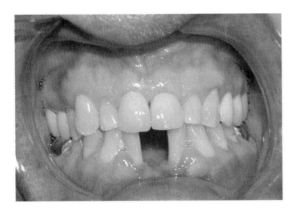

FIG. 10.12   Note significant bone shrinkage where two lower teeth have been removed.

- **Collapse of Facial Form:** Although not as severe as the facial changes caused by loss of all teeth, losing a few teeth also produces a sunken facial appearance. Teeth adjacent to the space move into peculiar positions. The appearance of a smile with a few missing teeth is considered unacceptable by most people (**FIG. 10.11**).

- **Bone Shrinkage:** When a few teeth are removed, the supporting bone shrinks from then on, leaving a defect in contour in that area (**FIG. 10.12**).

- **Reduced Eating Efficiency:** Reduced eating efficiency is directly related to the number of teeth lost. After removal of many teeth, chewing efficiency is reduced significantly, but removal of one or a few teeth does not seem to cause major loss of chewing effectiveness. The smile's appearance is the most neg-

ative characteristic caused by removal of a few teeth.

If you have had numerous teeth removed, you have the following alternatives:

A. **Conventional Fixed Partial Denture (Bridge):** A conventional fixed partial denture attaches to the natural teeth remaining in the mouth. You cannot remove this prosthesis (p. 149).

B. **Conventional Removable Partial Denture:** A conventional removable partial denture rests on, but does not attach to, the remaining teeth in the mouth. You can remove this prosthesis at will for cleaning (p. 162).

C. **Place Implants and Construct a Removable Partial Denture:** Place implants and construct a *removable partial denture* that rests on, and is retained by, the implants and the remaining natural teeth. You can remove this prosthesis at will for cleaning (p. 70).

D. **Place Implants and Construct a Fixed Partial Denture:** Place implants and construct a *fixed partial denture* that is attached to implants alone or to implants and the remaining teeth. You cannot remove this prosthesis (p. 71).

E. **Do Nothing:** If you elect to do nothing, your remaining natural teeth will continue to move, and your bite will usually collapse and degenerate further. This is not a good alternative in most cases for more than a short time.

3. One of Your Natural Teeth Has Been Removed

Two situations exist after the removal of one tooth:

A. *An unsightly appearance is created when a front tooth is removed* (**FIG. 10.13**). This condition is unacceptable in most societies, and it usually influences people to seek treatment. When a back tooth is removed, the cosmetic appearance is not observed, and patients may not be motivated to have an examination of the affected area until the following changes have occurred:

B. *The movement of surrounding teeth and collapse of the bite* (**FIG. 10.14**) *occur*

Implant Dentistry

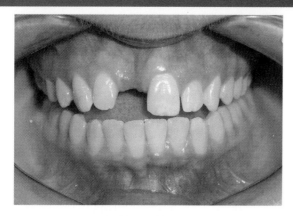

FIG. 10.13   You probably wouldn't like to have this smile. Simple repairs are available.

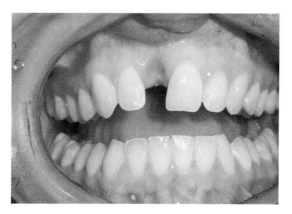

FIG. 10.14   The teeth next to the space moved after the tooth was extracted, creating a difficult rehabilitative challenge.

rapidly. Often within weeks the surrounding and opposing teeth start to collapse toward the space that was created by the tooth removal, making an acceptable replacement difficult. The contacting areas of teeth near the space may open, and food may become impacted between the teeth.

If you have one missing tooth, you have the following alternatives:

(1) **Conventional Fixed Bridge.** A conventional fixed bridge attaches to the teeth adjacent to the space. You cannot remove this prosthesis (p. 149).

(2) **Removable Partial Denture.** A removable partial denture fills the missing tooth space and allows an improved appearance and nearly normal function (p. 162).

(3) **Implant Followed by Crown (Cap).** Place an implant and place a crown (cap) over the implant head, thereby creating near optimal function and appearance. You cannot remove this crown (cap) (p. 72).

WHAT YOUR DENTIST CAN DO
Treatment Available

Replacing teeth with implants and overlying artificial teeth may be classified broadly into the following major categories: (1) replacement of all of the natural teeth when the patient has no teeth; (2) partial replacement of a few or several missing natural teeth, using remaining natural teeth to complete the normal number of teeth in the mouth; and (3) replacement of one tooth only. Replacements for missing teeth may be constructed to be removable by patients or fixed permanently into the mouth. Under certain conditions, all three of the replacements described may be attached to implants. The following paragraphs describe and illustrate the types of treatment (prostheses) that are available to be placed over dental implants.

1. Implants and Complete Dentures, Removable

Implants followed by complete removable dentures are among the most highly acceptable replacements for conventional complete dentures available. In this type of treatment, prostheses that appear to be similar to standard dentures are held in place by small spheres **(FIG. 10.15)** or bars with clips that fit over them **(FIG. 10.16)**, or other attachments such as magnets **(FIG. 10.17)**. The dentures are removable and must be taken out of the mouth frequently to clean the dentures, implants, and oral soft tissue.

A. **Advantages:** Placing implants and complete removable dentures allows good to excellent stability of the dentures when chewing, as well as high retention of the dentures in the mouth. It is one of the easiest and least expensive alternatives for significant improvement of the effectiveness of complete dentures. The cost

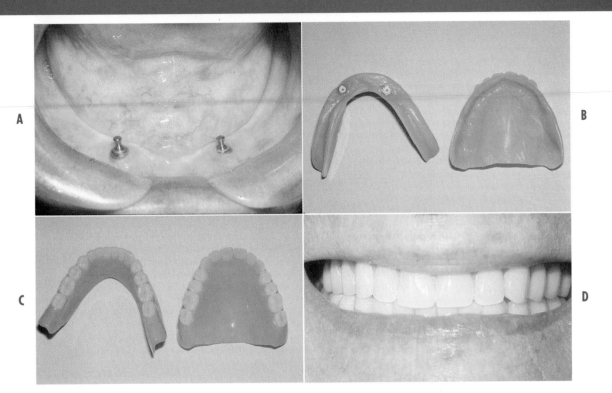

FIG. 10.15   **A,** Implants with small spherical heads on them. **B,** Artificial dentures. Note two rubber retentive washers in the lower denture. **C,** The chewing side of the dentures appears to be normal. **D,** The patient looks excellent and chews well.

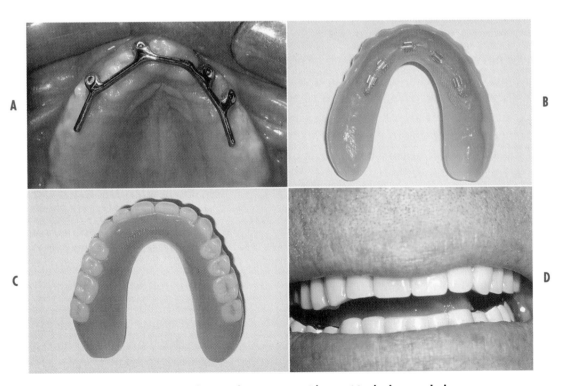

FIG. 10.16   **A,** Four implants in the upper jaw with a semicircular bar attached. **B,** Gold alloy clips inside the denture attach to the bar. **C,** The upper denture has no palate. **D,** The patient looks well and chews normally.

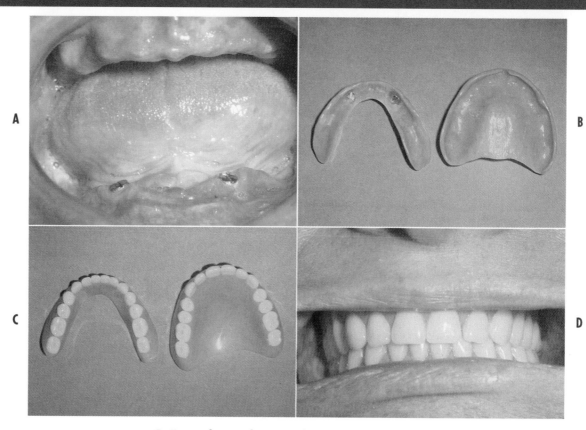

FIG. 10.17 **A,** Two implants with "magnet keepers" in them. **B,** Dentures, with two magnets in the lower one. **C,** Denture appearance is normal otherwise. **D,** The patient has a greatly improved, beautiful artificial dentition.

of this alternative is among the least expensive of implant-supported tooth replacements. It is also relatively easy to repair in the event of breakage. The appearance of this tooth replacement can be excellent, because it replaces both teeth and gums well.

B. **Disadvantages:** Removable dentures must be taken out of the mouth several times each day for cleaning; they are not fixed into place similar to natural teeth. The patient does not have the feeling of natural teeth. Because the dentures must be taken out frequently, there is the chance of breakage by dropping or aggressive cleaning.

C. **Risks:** Surgical risks are explained on p. 92. After the implants have been integrated into place and the dentures made, the risks are low. Occasionally, implants fail in service, but if this occurs they can usually be replaced. Few prostheses fail before serving for a

significant number of years, at which time they can be replaced or repaired with relative ease. If an implant fails, it can be replaced, and the prosthesis can be repaired or remade.

D. **Alternatives:** Patients have the following alternatives:
1. Make new conventional dentures without implants (p. 163)
2. Reline or rebase your current old dentures without implants (p. 161)
3. Modify your mouth surgically and make new conventional dentures without implants (p. 97)
4. Place implants and a fixed (nonremovable for you) denture over the implants (p. 69)
5. Do nothing.

E. **Costs:** The cost of dentures made without any implants is moderate. Adaptation of dentures to implants with heads such as small spheres (see **FIG. 10.15**) is inexpensive, while adaptation of dentures to a "bar-and-clip" arrangement (see **FIG. 10.16**) or other attachment (see **FIG. 10.17**) is more difficult and expensive. Cost of the bar and clip or other attachments adds cost to the treatment. Nevertheless, these three types of therapy provide the lowest cost for an implant-supported and retained prosthesis.

F. **Result of Nontreatment:** If you do nothing, you will continue with the same condition, and further bone and soft tissue degeneration probably will continue until you are forced to obtain therapy for your condition.

2. Implants and Complete Denture, Fixed

(**FIGS. 10.18 and 10.19**). When possible, placement of implants followed by a complete fixed denture is among the best available treatments for persons without any remaining natural teeth. However, some persons without teeth cannot have this therapy because of the lack of remaining bone support, and it is the most expensive of the treatments for persons without teeth.

A. **Advantages:** This treatment looks, feels, and functions in a manner similar to natural teeth. The prostheses stay in the mouth all the time and are removable only by a dentist. Almost no one is dissatisfied with this therapy when it is accomplished properly.

B. **Disadvantages:** There are very few disadvantages compared with other alternatives. However, the treatment is difficult, time-consuming, and expensive, and the patient must have follow-up maintenance every several months to ensure that it is functioning in an acceptable manner.

C. **Risks:** Other than the normal surgical risks (p. 92), there are few risks to this therapy. The denture can be broken, and it will wear out eventually, requiring repair or replacement. Very infrequently, an implant may become infected and require removal, necessitating replacement of the implant and remaking of the prosthesis. The risks described do not occur frequently.

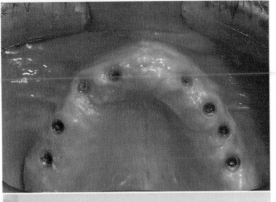

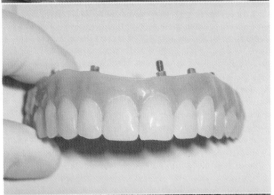

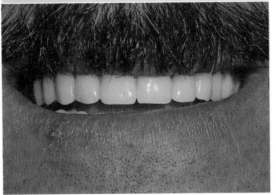

FIG. 10.18   A, Eight implants in upper jaw. **B,** Fixed detachable prosthesis (denture) can be removed only by dentist. **C,** Upper prosthesis screwed into edentulous upper jaw (no natural teeth present).

D. **Alternatives:** Patients have the following alternatives:
1. Make new conventional dentures without implants (p. 163)
2. Reline or rebase your old dentures without implants (p. 161)
3. Modify your mouth surgically and make new conventional dentures without implants (p. 97)
4. Place implants and a denture (removable for you) retained and supported by the implants (p. 66).
5. Do nothing.

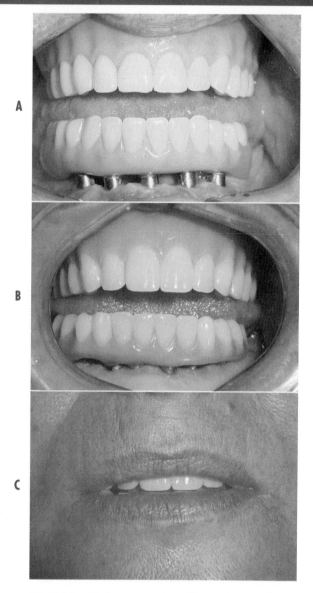

FIG. 10.19   **A,** Lower prosthesis (denture) screwed onto five implants. Space between gums and prosthesis is elective, does not show in normal conversation or smiling, and allows easy cleaning. **B,** Similar prosthesis, with less space present between prosthesis and gums. For chewing, such a prosthesis is as good as or better than natural teeth. **C,** Lower lip covers any space, even in the most animated mouth movements.

E. **Cost:** This therapy is several times more expensive than any other alternative for persons without teeth. However, almost all persons receiving it feel that the result justifies the cost.

F. **Result of Nontreatment:** If you do nothing, you will continue with the same condition, and it is predictable that further bone and soft tissue degeneration will continue until you are forced to obtain therapy for your condition.

3. Implants and Partial Dentures, Removable

(FIG. 10.20). When some natural teeth remain, implants may be placed in the positions where natural teeth are missing, and a partial denture can rest on the implants only or on the implants and the natural teeth.

A. **Advantages:** This treatment is less expensive than placing a fixed prosthesis on the implants, and it often allows a better appearance for the tooth and gum replacements than a fixed prosthesis does. It is more repairable than a fixed prosthesis. If a fixed prosthesis is preferred at a later time, the implants can be used for the fixed prosthesis.

B. **Disadvantages:** The only significant disadvantage is that the denture is removable by the patient and can be lost or broken while out of the mouth.

C. **Risks:** Other than the normal surgical risks (p. 92), this therapy is relatively risk-free, except that the denture can break or wear out. Infrequently, an implant may fail, requiring replacement and repair, or remaking of the denture.

D. **Alternatives:** Patients have the following alternatives:

1. Make a new conventional removable partial denture (p. 162)
2. If enough teeth remain, make a conventional fixed prosthesis, without implants (p. 149)
3. Reline or rebase your old removable partial denture without implants (p. 161)
4. Place implants and a fixed prosthesis retained and supported by the implants and not removable by you (p. 71)
5. Do nothing.

E. **Cost:** This therapy is less expensive than implants and a fixed prosthesis, but significantly more expensive than conventional removable partial dentures.

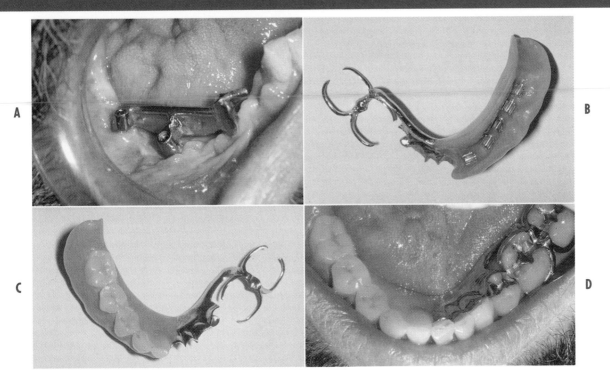

FIG. 10.20   **A,** Accident victim with three implants and bar in lower jaw. **B,** Lower removable partial denture. Note gold alloy clips to hold prosthesis (denture) in place. **C** and **D,** Lower prostheses both in and out of mouth appear normal but chew with excellent stability.

F. **Result of Nontreatment:** Natural teeth will continue to move, the bite will continue to collapse, and chewing efficiency will remain reduced.

4. Implants and Partial Dentures, Fixed

(FIG. 10.21). Implants and partial fixed dentures have many variations, most of which are among the most acceptable and successful in dentistry. These tooth replacements are screwed or cemented into place on the underlying implants, and they function and appear to be almost identical to natural teeth.

A. **Advantages:** These tooth replacements appear and feel very similar to natural teeth. They stay in place all the

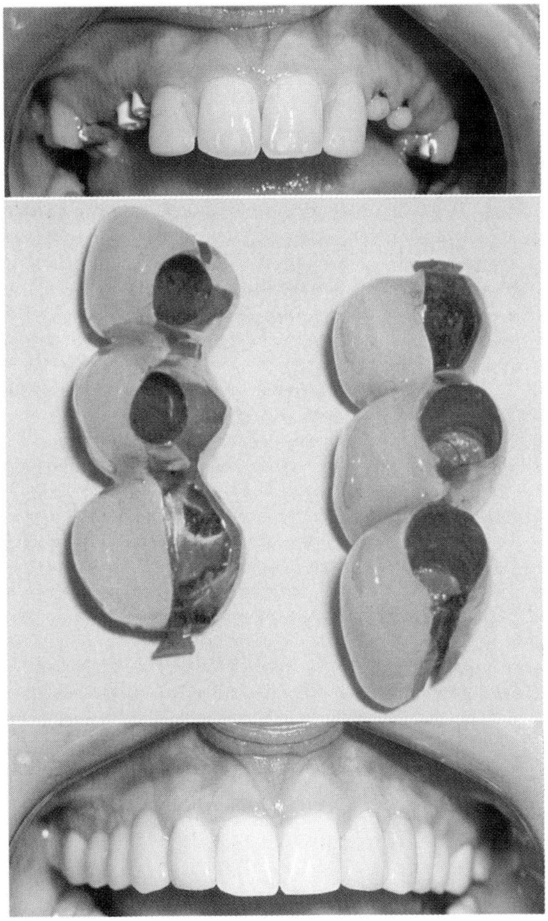

FIG. 10.21   **A,** Four implants in patient's upper jaw. **B,** Prosthesis (fixed denture) constructed to fit to both implants and natural teeth. They will be cemented into the mouth. **C,** Completed upper rehabilitation is beautiful and as functional as natural teeth.

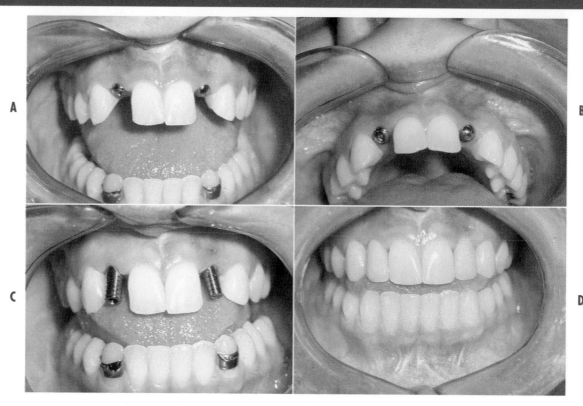

FIG. 10.22   A and B, Two implants were placed in upper jaw and allowed to heal for about 6 months with temporary denture in place. **C,** Abutment heads placed on implants, ready for dentist's contouring. **D,** Crowns (caps) cemented into place are undetectable!

time and are cleaned as though they were natural teeth.

B. **Disadvantages:** Fixed tooth replacements over implants are more expensive than removable ones, and when repair is necessary, it is more difficult than for removable replacements.

C. **Risks:** Other than the normal surgical risks of implants (p. 92), there are very few risks for the tooth replacement portion. Pieces of material can fracture from the fixed prosthesis, requiring repair or replacement. If an implant fails, the fixed prosthesis usually must be replaced.

D. **Alternatives:** If enough natural teeth remain:
1. Make a new removable partial denture, without implants (p. 162)
2. Make a conventional fixed bridge, without implants (p. 149)
3. Place implants and a removable partial denture, supported by the teeth and/or implants (p. 70)
4. Reline or rebase your old removable partial denture (p. 161)
5. Do nothing.

E. **Cost:** Fixed partial dentures over implants are more expensive than removable partial dentures over implants.

F. **Result of Nontreatment:** Natural teeth will continue to move, the bite will continue to collapse, and chewing efficiency will remain reduced.

5. Single Implant With a Crown (Cap)
(FIG. 10.22). This tooth replacement is very close to matching all the characteristics of a natural tooth.

A. **Advantages:** Adjacent teeth are not involved at all. The tooth feels and looks like a normal tooth.

B. **Disadvantages:** The cost of the implant and crown (cap) is relatively high and usually often equals the cost of a fixed bridge involving the two adjacent teeth.

C. **Risks:** Other than the normal surgical risks (p. 92), there are very few other potential problems. As with natural teeth, there is the possibility of breaking the crown (cap) portion on a hard piece of food or in an accident. Very infrequently the implant may fail, requiring that the procedure be repeated.

D. **Alternatives:** Patients have the following alternatives:
   1. Conventional or conservative fixed bridge involving adjacent teeth (p. 149)
   2. Conventional all-plastic or metal and plastic removable partial denture, replacing the missing tooth (p. 162)
   3. Reline, repair, or rebase an existing removable partial denture (p. 161)
   4. Do nothing.

E. **Cost:** The cost of replacing a single tooth, including the implant and the crown (cap), is up to three times the cost of placing a single crown (cap) on a natural tooth.

F. **Result of Nontreatment:** Natural teeth will continue to move, the bite will continue to collapse, continued bone loss will occur, and chewing efficiency will be impaired slightly.

SUMMARY

Although expensive, dental implants are one of the best treatment alternatives for people with many missing teeth, and often the only way to allow people without any teeth to chew well. Implants provide an alternative therapy for persons with only a few missing teeth. Implants have now had many years of clinical research and observation. When placed and maintained properly, they allow tooth and gum replacements that appear natural and function almost as effectively as natural teeth.

Implant Dentistry

CHAPTER 11

Occlusion

Your Bite, Temporomandibular Joints, Temporomandibular Dysfunction

Until recent years the area of occlusion in dentistry has not been emphasized. Therefore, many dentists have not been involved with treatment of people with occlusion problems. As a rule, the specialty most involved with movement of teeth to provide acceptable occlusion is orthodontics. Other areas of dentistry, including prosthodontics, periodontics, oral surgery, and general dentistry, are more involved with the condition commonly called *temporomandibular dysfunction* (TMD) or *temporomandibular joints* (TMJ) in the lay literature.

Currently, TMD is used most often to describe the syndrome (or disease), while TMJ is used to describe the anatomy of the specific location. This chapter is primarily concerned with TMD, whereas moving of teeth into proper function and appearance is included in the chapter on orthodontics (p. 99).

Your skeletal size is partially formed before your teeth erupt. As the primary (baby) teeth or permanent teeth erupt into the mouth one by one, the upper and lower teeth occlude (come together) in a haphazard way in direct relation to tooth size, size of the upper and lower jaws, relation of the jaw joints in the head, relation of jaws to one another, health of the patient, any oral habits, and numerous other factors. If all the factors are related in the manner that nature intended, the teeth will occlude (come together) correctly. If one or more of the factors is incorrect, malocclusion (incorrect bite) may be present, teeth may appear crooked and irregular, and the bite will be abnormal.

Other factors may cause a poor bite, including mixed genetics of various races; improper development of the jawbones; accidental trauma to the mouth; dental fillings, bridges and dentures; diseases such as arthritis; and other conditions.

Does a poor bite automatically stimulate a jaw dysfunction, pain, and jaw joint degeneration? No. However, one of the conditions that has been associated with TMD is a malaligned bite. This subject deserves an entire chapter because it has caused significant distress among patients, continual discussion by the lay press, and, most importantly, confusion among patients and all categories of health practitioners. Because some dentists do not treat occlusion, you may want to initiate the discussion of your specific problems with your general dentist. Referrals may be made to another general dentist; a prosthodontist; a periodontist; an oral surgeon; an ear, nose, and throat specialist; a chiropractor; or a physical therapist.

This chapter discusses clinical conditions that you can observe, as well as the treatment that your health practitioner can provide.

WHAT YOU SEE OR FEEL

Conditions, Signs or Symptoms Related to Occlusion, or Temporomandibular Dysfunction

1. Pain in the Head (Headaches), Neck, Shoulders
Often, unstimulated pain in the head, neck, and shoulders may be muscle dysfunction related to malaligned occlusion. This syndrome

is described as temporomandibular dysfunction (TMD). Innumerable causes are related to head and neck pain, and patients are advised to contact their dentist as soon as possible before making any conclusions, to confirm that the pain they are experiencing may or may not be related to occlusion (bite).

Pain related to occlusion and jaws is most common in the following locations: sides of head (temples), sides of lower jaw (cheeks), lateral sides of neck, back of head, top of shoulders, and upper back. Pain in one or all of these locations may be present at the same time. Usually, head pain (headaches) is not related to the jaws if it is in the eyes, nose, forehead, or top of the head. If pain is present in these locations, you probably do not have a jaw problem. Numerous diagnostic methods may be necessary to confirm that the pain is related to the jaw. Although there are many sophisticated treatment methods for muscle pain (headache) related to occlusion (bite), the simple, more common treatments, listed below, are emphasized in this book.

  A. Occlusal splint (bite splint) (p. 79)
  B. Occlusal equilibration (bite adjustment) (p. 78)
  C. Physical therapy (p. 80)
  D. Muscle relaxants (p. 78)
  E. Transcutaneous electrical neurostimulation (TENS) (p. 81)
  F. Hot or cold packs (p. 77)
  G. Do nothing

2. Clicking or Popping Jaw Joints

On movement of your jaw, you may feel or hear a "click" or "pop" on opening, closing, or both. This sound may be loud enough to attract the attention of other people, but it may be slight enough that only you are aware of it. Pain may or may not be associated with the sound. You may stimulate the pop by various movements of your mouth, or by chewing in ways that place stress on your jaw. A click without pain may not be a problem, but a click with pain usually signals that some problem is present. The usual conservative therapy for jaw joint clicking includes one or more of the following treatments:

  A. Occlusal splint (bite splint) (p. 79)
  B. Occlusal equilibration (bite adjustment) (p. 78)
  C. Physical therapy (p. 80)
  D. Muscle relaxants (p. 78)
  E. Transcutaneous electrical neurostimulation (TENS) (p. 81)
  F. Orthodontics (p. 80)
  G. Do nothing

3. Grinding or Grating Sound in Jaw Joints (Crepitus)

After months to years of mild jaw dysfunction and/or presence of other conditions such as an accident or arthritis, a grinding ("gravel") sound in the jaw joints may occur. This condition usually indicates some breakdown of the jaw joints that may or may not have been associated with the occlusion (bite). When this sound occurs, the possibility for successful, simple, conservative treatment is reduced. However, the sequence of therapy for grinding or grating jaw joints varies from relatively simple to complex. Any or all of the following treatments may be used:

  A. Occlusal splint (bite splint) (p. 79)
  B. Occlusal equilibration (bite adjustment) (p. 78)
  C. Physical therapy (muscle exercises) (p. 80)
  D. Muscle relaxants (p. 78)
  E. Transcutaneous electrical neurostimulation (TENS) (p. 81)
  F. Surgery on the temporomandibular joints (p. 81)
  G. Oral rehabilitation (rebuilding the teeth to a new occlusion [bite] with crowns [caps], fillings, bridges, etc.) (p. 79)
  H. Orthodontics (moving teeth to establish a new occlusion [bite]) (p. 80)
  I. Do nothing

4. Can't Open Jaw Or Can't Close Jaw

Occasionally the bones, ligaments, and muscles that make up the mechanism of the jaw joints become malaligned, and, as a result, the jaw locks open or closed. This can be painful as well as frustrating. Frequently, your dentist can assist the jaw to open with simple

Occlusion

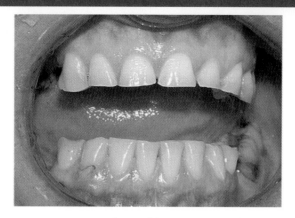

FIG. 11.1   Worn teeth caused by excessive tooth grinding, bruxism, or clenching.

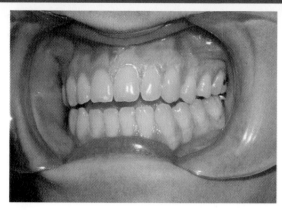

FIG. 11.2   Loose teeth caused by excessive contact on one or more teeth. Observe premature contact of teeth in back of mouth.

manipulations in the dental office, but more often other treatment is required. One or more of the following treatment methods will probably be used:

 A. Physical therapy muscle exercises (p. 80)
 B. Transcutaneous electrical neurostimulation (TENS) (p. 81)
 C. Muscle relaxants (p. 78)
 D. Occlusal splint (bite splint) (p. 79)
 E. Occlusal equilibration (bite adjustment) (p. 78)
 F. Do nothing

5. Teeth Visibly Worn From Bruxism or Clenching

At least one fourth to one third of the world population grinds their teeth excessively, thereby wearing tooth structure beyond normal expectations **(Fig. 11.1)**. This activity is called *bruxism* or *clenching*. During the first years of life this wear usually goes undetected, but soon it is evident, and concern is expressed. In the later stages of this problem, pain or even tooth death is caused by the wear. If you brux or clench your teeth excessively, you have the following potential treatment options, directly related to the severity of the condition as observed by your dentist:

 A. Occlusal splint (bite splint) (p. 79)
 B. Occlusal equilibration (bite adjustment) (p. 78)

 C. Oral rehabilitation (rebuilding the teeth to a new occlusion [bite] with crowns [caps], fillings, bridges, etc.) (p. 79)
 D. Removable partial denture made to cover the chewing surfaces (p. 162)
 E. Hypnosis to assist in slowing or stopping the bruxism (p. 77)
 F. Do nothing

6. Teeth Loose (Primary or Secondary Occlusal Trauma)

The occlusion (bite) may make teeth loose by overstressing them (primary occlusal trauma) **(Fig. 11.2)**, or the teeth may have reduced bone support from periodontal disease (gum and bone disease) (p. 129), and excess biting load can loosen them (secondary occlusal trauma). If the teeth are loose and the bone and gums are sound, the following therapy is indicated:

 A. Occlusal equilibration (bite adjustment) (p. 78)
 B. Occlusal splint (bite splint) (p. 79)
 C. Do nothing

If the bone and gums are weakened and the teeth are loose, the following treatment is indicated:

 A. Periodontal therapy (p. 135)
 B. Occlusal equilibration (bite adjustment) (p. 78)
 C. Occlusal splint (bite splint) (p. 79)
 D. Splinting teeth (p. 127)
 E. Do nothing

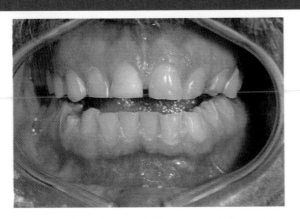

FIG. 11.3   Malocclusion; teeth do not meet in front of mouth.

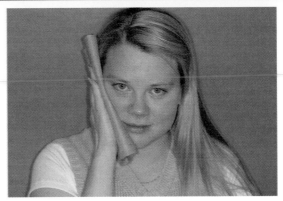

FIG. 11.4   Hot or cold packs for head and neck pain.

7. Teeth Do Not Occlude (Meet) Properly

You may not be able to chew well because your occlusion (bite) is incorrect **(Fig. 11.3)**. This condition is usually related to malpositioning of the teeth in the dental arch, or to a discrepancy between your tooth size and your jaw size (teeth are too large or too small for the jaws). You have the following treatment alternatives:

A. Orthodontics (move teeth) (p. 80)

B. Oral rehabilitation (rebuilding the teeth to a new occlusion [bite] with crowns [caps], fillings, bridges, etc.) (p. 79)

C. Orthognathic surgery (p. 95)

D. Occlusal equilibration (bite adjustment) (p. 78)

E. Do nothing

WHAT YOUR DENTIST CAN DO

Treatment Available

1. Hot or Cold Packs (Fig. 11.4)

A. **Advantages:** Placing hot or cold packs on the area of involvement is simple, easy, fast, and inexpensive and can be moderately effective.

B. **Disadvantages:** Hot or cold packs do not cure the disease; they only make it feel better for a while. This will allow other therapy to continue at the same time because it reduces pain. Placement of heat can become a habit, and its use should be restricted to a limited time.

C. **Risks:** No risk is involved unless used excessively. Soft-tissue damage can occur from overuse of hot packs.

D. **Alternatives:** Muscle-relaxing drugs (p. 78), physical therapy (p. 80), pain-reducing drugs, and transcutaneous electrical neurostimulation (TENS) (p. 81) application are alternatives.

E. **Cost:** Little cost is involved if ice in a plastic bag or hot, moist towels are used. Commercially available hot or cold packs are moderately priced.

F. **Result of Nontreatment:** The condition will continue to be painful with some limited function, but it may also disappear without treatment after a short period of rest.

2. Hypnosis for Occlusal (Bite) Problems

A. **Advantages:** Hypnosis can help to reduce or eliminate grinding or clenching of teeth, headaches, and other problems in a relatively simple, painless manner at a moderate cost. It is useful in helping to control many physical conditions.

B. **Disadvantages:** Hypnosis is effective for many but not all people. It is relatively time-consuming and requires the cooperation and acceptance of the patient. Only a small percentage of health practitioners include hypnosis in their practices, and finding one who does will demand effort on the patient's part.

Occlusion

C. **Risks:** Contrary to many public opinions of hypnosis, the patient is in complete control at all times. There are no risks with professionally managed hypnosis.

D. **Alternatives:** Hypnosis is an alternative therapy, and most of the other treatments listed in this chapter can be substituted for it, including drugs (p. 78), occlusal splint (bite splint) (p. 79), occlusal equilibration (bite adjustment) (p. 78), physical therapy (p. 80), and hot and cold packs (p. 77), among others. Often, these other therapies are included with hypnosis.

E. **Cost:** Although not as expensive as surgery, oral rehabilitation, or some other treatments, the cost of hypnosis is moderate, and it requires payment to the practitioner for the significant time involvement necessary.

F. **Result of Nontreatment:** The condition being treated would continue to require other therapy described in this chapter.

3. Muscle-Relaxant Drugs

A. **Advantages:** Discomfort caused by tense muscles will be reduced rapidly in most cases, and limited normal function usually follows soon.

B. **Disadvantages:** Most of these medications cause a feeling of tiredness, limiting physical and mental activity and causing relaxation of other body muscles also.

C. **Risks:** All drugs have some possible side effects and allergenic potential. If used for temporomandibular dysfunction, these medications should be limited in duration of use and dosage.

D. **Alternatives:** Hot and cold packs (p. 77), physical therapy (p. 80), pain-reducing drugs, and TENS application are alternatives.

E. **Cost:** Moderate cost should be expected for short-term use.

F. **Result of Nontreatment:** The same pain or limitation of movement will continue unless other therapy is provided.

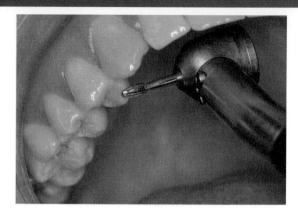

FIG. 11.5   Occlusal (bite) adjustment.

4. Occlusal Equilibration (Bite Adjustment) (Fig. 11.5)

A. **Advantages:** Bite adjustment removes slight amounts of previously placed crowns (caps), bridges, or incorrectly unworn enamel of the teeth from the chewing surfaces, to provide contact of the teeth all at once. When the upper and lower teeth meet at one time, the muscle tenseness and pain often disappear. The technique is simple, logical, and painless under normal conditions, and it corrects the bite imbalance immediately.

B. **Disadvantages:** Small amounts of tooth structure or dental filling material must be removed to balance the bite. Some may think of this as a disadvantage. However, the negative condition will not heal itself. It is similar to the tires of a car being out of balance; they will stay out of balance until they are altered mechanically.

C. **Risks:** Occasionally, fillings, crowns (caps), or bridges may be adjusted to balance the bite. If this is the case, these restorations must be repaired. An experienced practitioner will have no difficulty with bite adjustment, and the risks are very low.

D. **Alternatives:** If the jaws are truly out of alignment because the teeth do not contact correctly, there are very few alternatives to bite equilibration, other than wearing a bite-correcting splint all of the time or remaking the tooth

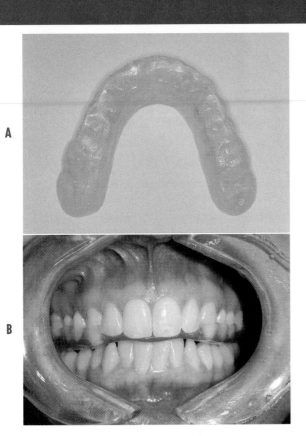

A

B

FIG. 11.6   **A and B, Occlusal (bite) splints.**

fillings, crowns (caps), and bridges to correct the relationship.

E. **Cost:** Bite adjustment has a moderate cost, equal to, more or less, the cost of one crown (cap).

F. **Result of Nontreatment:** The condition being treated will continue and/or worsen.

5. Occlusal Splint (Bite Splint) (Fig. 11.6)

A. **Advantages:** Wearing a bite splint of various types is reversible since it can be removed from the mouth, and the therapy is very effective. Splints direct the teeth to come together in the correct position or open the bite, placing biting force on the front teeth, relieving muscle stress. They also protect the remaining tooth structure from harm caused by excessive grinding, since the splint is worn by the opposing teeth.

B. **Disadvantages:** The pain relief brought about by a splint lasts only while the splint is worn. When the splint is removed for a significant period, the pain

often returns. Occlusal equilibration (bite adjustment) is usually needed after the splint has caused a reduction in pain to make the teeth occlude (come together) in the same jaw position developed by the splint. Splints wear out after a few years because they are usually softer than the opposing tooth structure into which they chew.

C. **Risks:** No risks are involved if the splint is used correctly. However, the splint can cause dental caries if the teeth are not cleaned well each day.

D. **Alternatives:** No treatment repositions the jaws or protects the teeth during bruxism as well or as inexpensively as an occlusal splint (bite splint). If an occlusal splint is indicated for your condition, it should be made.

E. **Cost:** The cost of an occlusal splint is moderate. It is usually no more than double the cost of one crown (cap), depending on the patient's needs.

F. **Result of Nontreatment:** Some other therapy will be necessary, or the condition will probably continue to worsen. A few cases get better with no treatment.

6. Oral Rehabilitation

Placement of crowns (caps) and bridges on all or most of the teeth is usually called an *oral rehabilitation* (Fig. 11.7). See Chapter 16 for details on crowns (caps) and bridges (p. 139).

A. **Advantages:** Oral rehabilitation usually establishes and stabilizes the correct relationship of the upper and lower jaws. Often the appearance of teeth and the smile can be upgraded significantly also.

B. **Disadvantages:** The cost of this procedure is high, and after a period of years, it will probably need to be redone because of wear and breakage. Crowns (caps) are usually used for an occlusal rehabilitation. Significant time is required for the therapy.

C. **Risks:** Oral rehabilitation can occasionally stimulate the need for endodontic (root canal) therapy in some teeth.

Occlusion

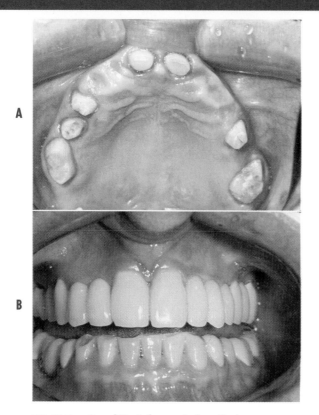

A

B

FIG. 11.7 A and **B,** Before and after. Oral rehabilitation rebuilds all of the occlusal (chewing) surfaces of the teeth.

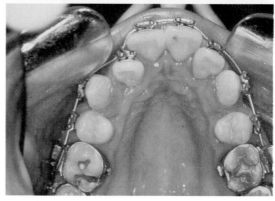

FIG. 11.8   Orthodontic therapy in progress, using brackets bonded to teeth. (From Viazis A: *Atlas of advanced orthodontics: a guide to clinical efficiency,* Philadelphia, 1998, WB Saunders.)

Also, there is no assurance that the rehabilitation will solve the jaw problem totally.

D. **Alternatives:** An occlusal splint (p. 79) can be worn indefinitely to develop and maintain an acceptable relationship of the upper and lower teeth and the proper alignment of the jaws.

E. **Cost:** Any of the oral rehabilitation methods are among the most expensive therapies in dentistry.

F. **Result of Nontreatment:** The condition being treated will continue to worsen.

7. Orthodontic Therapy (Moving Teeth)

Orthodontic therapy is indicated occasionally for occlusal dysfunction **(Fig. 11.8).** See Chapter 13 for a detailed discussion of orthodontics (p. 99).

A. **Advantages:** When indicated, orthodontic therapy is used to move the natural teeth to the correct position to stabilize the relationship of the jaws.

B. **Disadvantages:** Several months to several years are required for orthodontic therapy. The teeth have various wires, brackets, or bands on them during treatment.

C. **Risks:** Any significant movement of teeth in adults can sometimes cause a need for irreversible conditions such as endodontics (root canal therapy), shortening of tooth roots by root resorption (degeneration), and other conditions. Additionally, there is no assurance that orthodontic therapy will solve all the occlusal conditions until after the tooth movement has been completed.

D. **Alternatives:** Occlusal rehabilitation, wearing occlusal splints (bite splints) indefinitely, and occlusal equilibration (bite adjustment) are some of the alternatives to orthodontic therapy.

E. **Cost:** The cost of this treatment is between the high cost of oral rehabilitation and the low cost of an occlusal splint.

F. **Result of Nontreatment:** The condition will continue until some other therapy is completed.

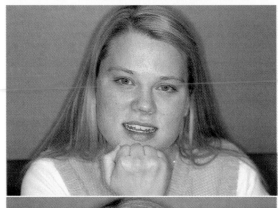

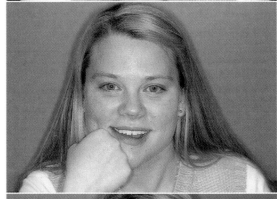

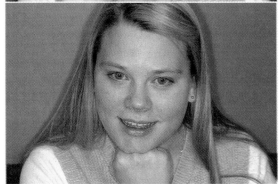

FIG. 11.9   A to C, Physical therapy using passive, stretching, and resistant exercises.

8. Physical Therapy (Fig. 11.9)

A. **Advantages:** Physical therapy is simple, relatively pain-free, inexpensive, and effective. When conducted properly, it is reversible and nondamaging.

B. **Disadvantages:** The exercises are often time consuming and may be somewhat painful. They require supervision at first for adequate understanding. The patient must have self-discipline.

C. **Risks:** Properly provided, physical therapy is not different from normal exercise. There are very few risks.

D. **Alternatives:** Some good, conservative alternatives are TENS therapy (p. 81), muscle relaxant drugs (p. 78), and pain-reducing medications.

E. **Cost:** Physical therapy has a relatively low cost compared with the other therapy methods described in this chapter.

F. **Result of Nontreatment:** The condition will usually continue to worsen.

9. Surgery of the Temporomandibular Joints

See Chapter 12 for a discussion of this area (p. 83).

A. **Advantages:** If conditions are severe enough for surgery to be suggested, the chances for success are good. Very few patients need surgery. Only about 1% to 5% of patients with jaw problems have a condition serious enough to require surgery.

B. **Disadvantages:** Some of these surgical procedures require several weeks for healing, are somewhat painful, and are relatively expensive. Sometimes the jaws are wired shut to allow healing for up to 6 weeks.

C. **Risks:** As with any surgery, there is the risk from anesthesia, unexpected negative surgical outcome, and inadvertent damage to other anatomical structures.

D. **Cost:** This therapy is among the more expensive treatment methods discussed in this chapter.

E. **Result of Nontreatment:** The condition will continue to worsen unless treated.

10. Transcutaneous Electrical Neurostimulation (TENS)

TENS involves a small electrical current applied to muscles, usually relaxing them easily and fast, thus relieving pain (Fig. 11.10).

A. **Advantages:** Muscle relaxation and pain relief.

B. **Disadvantages:** TENS is time consuming and requires patient understanding and cooperation for success. Further therapy is usually necessary.

Occlusion

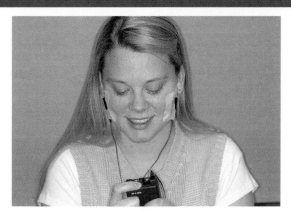

FIG. 11.10 **Transcutaneous electrical neurostimulation (TENS) for head and neck pain.**

C. **Risks:** Properly administered, TENS has almost no risks, but it cannot be used in some situations such as in persons who have pacemakers or in pregnant women.

D. **Alternatives:** Acceptable alternatives are physical therapy (p. 80), muscle relaxant drugs (p. 78), occlusal splints (bite splints) (p. 79), and pain-reducing drugs.

E. **Cost:** TENS therapy has a low cost.

F. **Result of Nontreatment:** The condition will usually continue to worsen unless treated.

SUMMARY

Occlusal (bite) problems are complex, confusing, and relatively difficult to treat. Opinions among practitioners vary widely, and a second or third opinion is suggested before treatment. Occlusal problems require very competent, experienced practitioners who are willing to work with others on the health care team. Patients need to be cooperative and accepting.

Diseases and Surgery Related to the Oral and Facial Areas

Many diseases in various parts of the body have oral implications. In fact, the mouth is a mirror of overall body health. Dentists can tell about general body health by looking in the mouth, observing the condition of the soft and hard tissues, and repeating the examination over a period of weeks or months for comparison. The condition of the teeth and the bone and gums that support them are dependent on numerous conditions, including hereditary factors, diet, oral hygiene, and overall health. You should consult your dentist or dental specialist about any conditions or diseases of the oral cavity or related structures. These practitioners are the most educated and experienced of all health practitioners with regard to that part of the body. In the event that your dentist does not recognize your oral condition, he or she will refer you to the appropriate practitioner for further observation.

Most of the oral conditions, except for dental caries (tooth decay), periodontal disease (gum and bone degeneration), and malocclusion (bad bite and crooked teeth), are generally classified into oral medicine or oral pathology. The specialists treating these remaining conditions are usually oral and maxillofacial surgeons, other specialists, or general dentists with interest in this area. A significant number of these conditions require surgery. A small recognized dental specialty, oral pathology, exists but oral pathologists accomplish primarily microscopic recognition of oral diseases as assistance for other dentists.

Most general dentists extract teeth when that procedure is required. However, oral and maxillofacial surgeons have additional education and experience in all surgical aspects of this portion of the body, and many dentists prefer to refer the more difficult procedures, tooth extractions, and other surgical needs to specialists. Your general dentist will judge whether your situation should be referred to an oral and maxillofacial surgeon.

Teeth serve a vital function in the human body, and extraction of teeth should be avoided just as vigorously as amputation of a finger, toe, or any other part of the body. Satisfactory replacement of teeth with artificial ones is difficult and expensive. Only if the entire procedure is done at a high level of quality and skill will the artificial result resemble and function as well as natural teeth. Many conditions described in this book list tooth extraction as an alternative, but it is strongly suggested that teeth be extracted only as a last option.

WHAT YOU SEE OR FEEL

Conditions, Signs, or Symptoms Related to Oral and Maxillofacial Surgery, Oral Pathology, or Oral Medicine

Some of the conditions discussed below have been listed in other chapters also, because their presence in a less severe form does not require surgery. In such cases you will be referred to the location in the book that describes the more conservative treatment.

1. Loose Teeth (Fig. 12.1): When you bite on your teeth, you feel movement, and when you grasp them with your fingers and apply

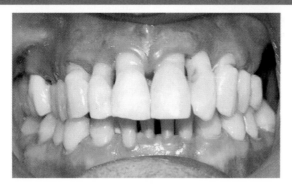

FIG. 12.1   Loose teeth caused by periodontal disease (bone and gum degeneration).

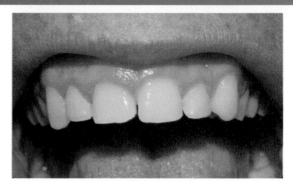

FIG. 12.2   Slightly broken tooth.

force, you can feel and see movement. Sometimes the looseness may be so severe that you feel that you could extract a tooth yourself or force it out by eating.

Several conditions cause loose teeth. The most common ones are described below:

- **Periodontal disease (degeneration of the jaw bones and gums) (p. 129):** Periodontal disease causes a reduction in the amount of bone support, and progresses to tooth loosening. This condition continues until it is stopped with help from a periodontist, general dentist, or dental hygienist; it will not heal itself. You have one or more of the following options:
  A. Scaling teeth (removal of hard deposits) (p. 134)
  B. Periodontal surgery (p. 135)
  C. Fixed prosthesis, Maryland Bridge (p. 152)
  D. Crowns (caps) splinted together (p. 146)
  E. Teeth splinted together by bonding with reinforced plastic (p. 127)
  F. Tooth extraction (p. 92) and artificial tooth replacements
- **Trauma (a blow to the teeth):** If you have had an injury to your teeth that has loosened but not broken one or more of them, the possibility for recovery is good. Usually the teeth will return to normal after a period of weeks, but some may require endodontics (root canal therapy) because of a dead pulp (nerve). Treatment options include the following:
  A. Pushing teeth back into place, avoiding

heavy chewing for a few weeks, and awaiting healing
  B. Splinting the teeth together by bonding with reinforced plastic until healing has occurred

Some teeth that have been repositioned after a severe blow require endodontics (root canal therapy). This is recognized by the patient or dentist because of continuing pain in the tooth over a period of weeks, and possible tooth discoloration. A few teeth that have received a blow bond to the bone and become ankylosed (solidly attached to the bone). These teeth may continue to function at an acceptable level; others resorb (degenerate). Tooth extraction is not usually indicated.

2. Gums Bleed Easily: Bleeding gums are described in the chapter on periodontics (gum and bone diseases) (p. 129). Usually this condition is a result of periodontal disease. Periodontal (gum) surgery may be possible (p. 135). Tooth extraction is the last and least desirable possibility.

3. Slightly Broken Tooth (Fig. 12.2): A break of the coronal portion of the tooth (tooth part that normally appears when you open your mouth) is usually repairable with relatively simple restorative methods (p. 142).

4. Moderately Broken Tooth (Fig. 12.3): If most of the coronal portion of the tooth is broken off, and the pulp (nerve) of the tooth is visible in the center of the tooth (it is red and may bleed), endodontics (root canal therapy) is usually required (p. 40), and a crown (cap) usually must be placed on the tooth.

5. Severely Broken Tooth (Fig. 12.4): Occasionally, teeth may be broken to the extent

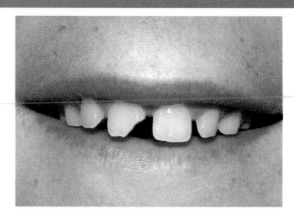

FIG. 12.3   Moderately broken tooth.

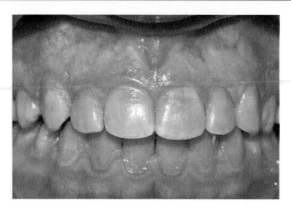

FIG. 12.5   Gray or pink teeth.

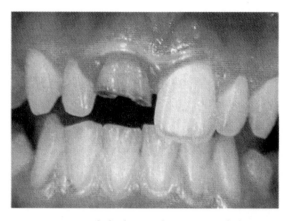

FIG. 12.4   Severely broken tooth requiring endodontics (root canal therapy). (From Tyldesley WR: *Colour atlas of orofacial diseases,* ed 2, St Louis, 1991, Mosby [Wolfe]. Copyright 1991 by WR Tyldesley.)

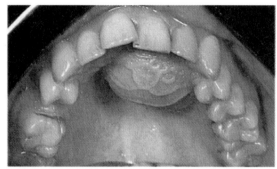

FIG. 12.6   Swelling in palate related to diseased tooth. (From Tyldesley WR: *Colour atlas of orofacial diseases,* ed 2, St Louis, 1991, Mosby [Wolfe]. Copyright 1991 by WR Tyldesley.)

that none of the coronal portion shows when you open your mouth. The root portion of the tooth may be visible below the gum line. If such a tooth can be saved, it almost always requires endodontic (root canal) therapy (p. 40), a reinforcement post, and an extensive crown (cap) (p. 146).

If the tooth has fractured vertically into the root (which is segregated into two portions), it almost always requires extraction and the necessary replacement procedures (p. 92). A few heroic bonding procedures may save the tooth.

6. Tooth Knocked Out of Mouth: A severe blow to the face and mouth can dislodge a tooth completely from the mouth. If this happens, try to find the tooth immediately. Place it in a cup of milk or in the mouth under the upper or lower lip. Find a dentist immediately, and have the dentist decide whether the tooth should be replanted into its socket. Such replanted teeth often become functional again. The longer the tooth remains out of the mouth, the less chance there is for success when it is replanted.

If the tooth is lost, or if replanting is considered unacceptable, the same replacement procedures for an extracted tooth are necessary (fixed prosthodontics, p. 139).

7. Tooth Appears Gray or Pink (Fig. 12.5): A gray tooth usually has a dead pulp (nerve) and requires endodontic (root canal) therapy (p. 40). A pink tooth may have an enlarged pulp (nerve) and may require endodontic (root canal) therapy (p. 40). In severe situations in which teeth appear gray or pink, extraction may be necessary (p. 92).

8. Swelling in the Jaws or Neck (Fig. 12.6): Swelling in the mouth, upper or lower jaw, or neck that has come on rapidly is probably associated with a diseased tooth. Treatment of

Oral and Maxillofacial Surgery

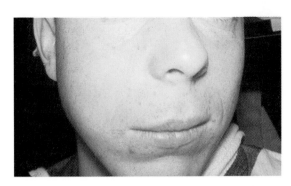

FIG. 12.7   **Slow swelling in face not related to diseased tooth.**

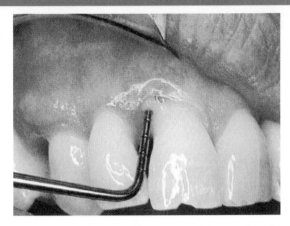

FIG. 12.9   **Oozing pus from gums caused by periodontal disease (bone and gum degeneration).** (From Tyldesley WR: *Colour atlas of orofacial diseases,* ed 2, St Louis, 1991, Mosby [Wolfe]. Copyright 1991 by WR Tyldesley.)

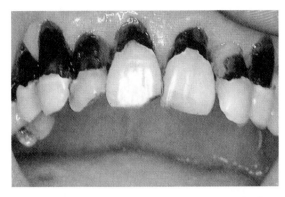

FIG. 12.8   **Decayed teeth, resulting in severe toothache when the person eats sweets.** (From Tyldesley WR: *Colour atlas of orofacial diseases,* ed 2, St Louis, 1991, Mosby [Wolfe]. Copyright 1991 by WR Tyldesley.)

the swelling probably requires drainage and endodontics (root canal therapy) on a specific tooth (p. 40). Severely diseased teeth that have caused swelling may require removal of one or more teeth (p. 92).

Swelling that slowly develops **(Fig. 12.7)** in the upper or lower jaws or the neck over a period of months or years is usually some form of tumor or cyst, and it should have professional observation as soon as the swelling is recognized. Such swellings are usually not associated with teeth, but they may require a biopsy (small piece of tissue to be observed under a microscope) (p. 91) and/or surgery for removal.

9. Pain in Tooth: A carious (decayed) tooth can cause pain **(Fig. 12.8)**, but it may re-

quire only a restoration (filling) or endodontics (root canal therapy) (p. 40) and a restoration (filling), or an extraction (p. 92). Pain in a tooth does not necessarily require an extraction.

10. Sensitivity to Pressure on a Specific Tooth: A pressure-sensitive tooth usually calls for endodontics (root canal therapy) (p. 40). However, the tooth may have had root canal therapy already and may need further endodontic treatment or extraction (p. 92). Pressure sensitivity can also be caused by a heavy occlusion (bite) (p. 74), excessive bruxism or clenching (grinding teeth) (p. 76), or a crack in the tooth (p. 142).

11. Pus Oozing From Gums (Fig. 12.9): Pus oozing from gums usually indicates teeth that are in the late stages of periodontal disease. Such teeth require either periodontal (gum and bone) surgery or tooth extraction.

12. Pimple Protruding From Gums (Fig. 12.10): A pimple on the gum usually indicates a dead pulp (nerve) of a tooth; the pimple provides an escape of pus from the root end of the tooth. Such teeth can usually be treated by endodontics (root canal therapy) (p. 40), apicoectomy (surgical removal of a small piece of tooth root and filling of the root canal on the root end) (p. 41), or, in extreme cases, extraction of the offending tooth (p. 92).

13. Decayed Teeth (Fig. 12.11): Dental caries (decay) whether small, medium, or large, can

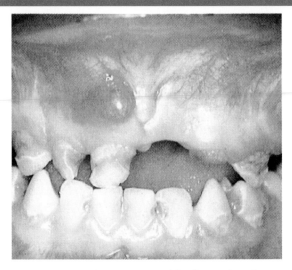

FIG. 12.10   Pimple on gum caused by diseased tooth. (From Tyldesley WR: *Colour atlas of orofacial diseases,* ed 2, St Louis, 1991, Mosby [Wolfe]. Copyright 1991 by WR Tyldesley.)

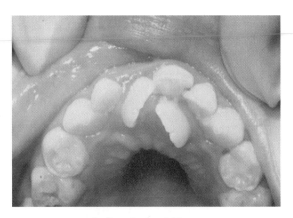

FIG. 12.12   Crooked teeth in a child, requiring extraction of primary (baby) teeth. (From Cameron A, Widmer R: *Handbook of pediatric dentistry,* London, 1997, Mosby-Wolfe.)

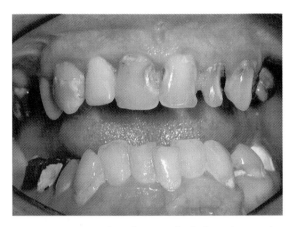

FIG. 12.11   Decayed teeth, most of which can be saved by restorations (fillings).

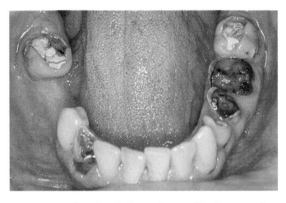

FIG. 12.13   Chronic pain in teeth caused by long-standing dental caries (decay).

usually be treated by simple restorations (fillings) (p. 170) or crowns (caps) (p. 146). Only long-neglected dental caries (decay) destroys teeth sufficiently to require extraction (p. 92).

14. Crooked Teeth (Fig. 12.12): Crooked teeth should be straightened by orthodontic therapy (p. 107). However, occasionally there are too many teeth for the size of the jaws, or the teeth are too large for the space present, and some teeth must be extracted before orthodontics can be accomplished.

15. Chronic Tooth Pain (Fig. 12.13): Long-standing chronic pain in a tooth requires definitive diagnosis. The tooth could have

deep dental caries (decay). It could have a dead pulp (nerve), requiring endodontics (root canal therapy) (p. 40). It may be cracked, requiring a crown (cap) (p. 146) and possibly root canal therapy. It could be that a previous root canal treatment has failed, requiring redoing of the root canal or extraction of the tooth. Chronic pain could also be the result of bruxism (grinding teeth).

16. Unerupted Teeth (Fig. 12.14): An impacted (unerupted) or partially erupted tooth can cause problems by developing various abnormal growing patterns that destroy surrounding bone, or by growing into the mouth

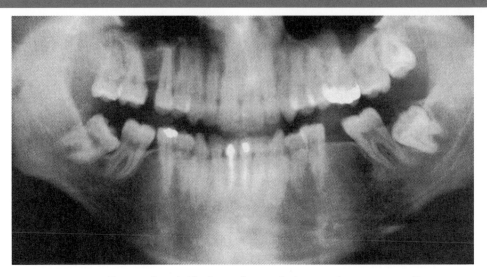

FIG. 12.14   **Unerupted teeth. The last molars on the lower arch cannot erupt.** (From McGowan DA: *An atlas of minor oral surgery: principles and practice*, ed 2, London, 1999, Martin Dunitz Ltd. Copyright 1999 by DA McGowan.)

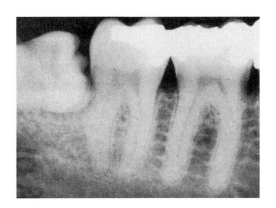

FIG. 12.15   **Impacted wisdom tooth that requires extraction.** (From McGowan DA: *An atlas of minor oral surgery: principles and practice*, ed 2, London, 1999, Martin Dunitz Ltd. Copyright 1999 by DA McGowan.)

in peculiar locations. Often an impacted tooth that could potentially erupt into the mouth for normal service can be stimulated to erupt by exposing it surgically (p. 127). An impacted tooth may require orthodontic treatment (movement) to push or pull it into place (p. 107). Occasionally an impacted tooth requires extraction because normal eruption cannot occur because of lack of space in the mouth or evidence of pathological (disease) activity present on the tooth. Sometimes an impacted tooth should be allowed to remain impacted. Third molars (wisdom teeth) that cannot erupt properly (Fig. 12.15) because of lack of space are often extracted. It is advis-

able to consult a few dentists or specialists before deciding on the proper treatment for impacted teeth.

17. Broken Jaw: Trauma to the face occasionally breaks the upper or lower jaw (maxilla or mandible) and associated bones. Oral and maxillofacial surgeons are usually the most appropriate specialists to set these bones, since these practitioners know the specific anatomy of the oral-facial area, and they know how the teeth should come together (occlude) better than any other specialists in the entire medical area.

18. Lower Jaw Too Far Forward or Too Far Backward (Fig. 12.16): Excellent surgical treatment is available for correction of jaws that do not meet the normal appearance standards or that do not function well. Lower or upper jaws may be moved forward or backward by orthognathic surgery (p. 95). Orthodontics (tooth movement) (p. 107) may be necessary as a part of this therapy.

19. Upper or Lower Jawbone Inadequate for Dentures (Fig. 12.17): Extraction of teeth causes loss of jawbone, and each year after tooth extraction the jawbone shrinks from $\frac{1}{16}$ to $\frac{1}{32}$ inch per year. Eventually the jawbone becomes inadequate to hold and support a denture. Numerous surgical procedures are available to add bulk to the bone by placement of artificial or real bone (ridge augmen-

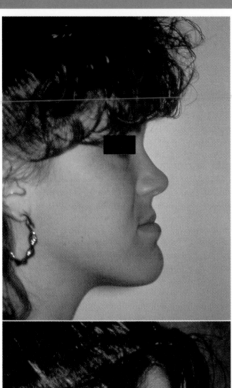

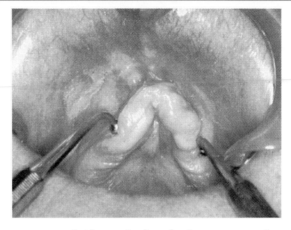

FIG. 12.17   Inadequate jawbone for denture construction requires surgery, bone rebuilding, and/or implants. (From Tyldesley WR: *Colour atlas of orofacial diseases*, ed 2, St Louis, 1991, Mosby [Wolfe]. Copyright 1991 by WR Tyldesley.)

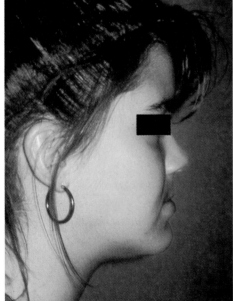

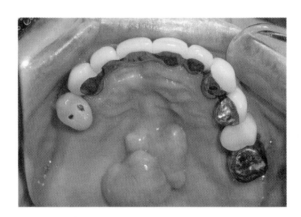

FIG. 12.18   Hard growths.

FIG. 12.16   Lower jaw requiring corrective surgery to reduce prominence of chin. (From Viazis A: *Atlas of advanced orthodontics: a guide to clinical efficiency*, Philadelphia, 1998, WB Saunders.)

tation) (p. 94). Additionally, the soft tissue on the bony ridge may be extended deeper into the jawbone (vestibuloplasty) to create greater space for the denture (p. 97). Jaws that have especially shrunken bone can often be changed significantly by the addition of two or more dental implants on which dentures may be placed (p. 70). Additional support and retention for shrunken jaws is created with this technique.

20. Jaw Joints Hurt or Jaw Muscles Ache: The so-called temporomandibular joint syndrome (TMJ), more accurately described as temporomandibular dysfunction (TMD), is more common than previously recognized. Sometimes this condition can be treated by conservative therapy, including occlusal (bite) splints (p. 79), muscle physical therapy (p. 80), or occlusal (bite) adjustment (p. 78). However, occasionally, degenerate jaw joints require surgery for proper correction (p. 95).

21. Hard Growths in Mouth (Fig. 12.18): Most hard projections in the mouth, called benign exostoses (bone growths), are not dangerous. They occur most commonly in the roof of the mouth, under the tongue, and on the upper jaw on the cheek side of the molars.

Oral and Maxillofacial Surgery

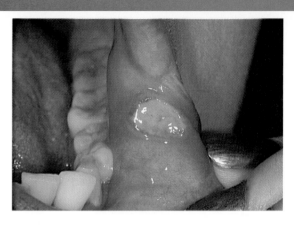

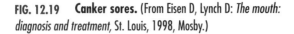

FIG. 12.19 **Canker sores.** (From Eisen D, Lynch D: *The mouth: diagnosis and treatment,* St. Louis, 1998, Mosby.)

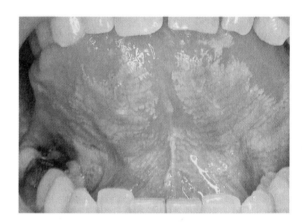

FIG. 12.20 **White spots under a patient's tongue demand professional consultation.** (From Tyldesley WR: *Colour atlas of orofacial diseases,* ed 2, St Louis, 1991, Mosby [Wolfe]. Copyright 1991 by WR Tyldesley.)

If these projections interfere with speech or eating, they may be removed; otherwise, they should be allowed to remain in place.

22. Cold Sores: Irritating sores occur on the lips of many people. They are caused by the herpesvirus and are nearly impossible to cure completely. Your dentist will be able to suggest numerous medications that assist in reducing both the occurrence and the severity of these frustrating lesions. They do not require surgery.

23. Canker Sores (Fig. 12.19): Ulcers occur in the mouths of many people on a consistent basis, located in sites of irritation or arising seemingly spontaneously. They are painful and limit speech and eating patterns. These lesions, of viral origin, are nearly impossible to prevent totally, but your dentist will be able to suggest several medications to limit their occurrence and reduce their severity. Canker sores do not require surgery.

24. Dry Mouth: Many body conditions, such as normal aging, salivary gland problems, numerous medications taken frequently, ra-

diation therapy or chemotherapy, can cause xerostomia (dry mouth). This condition influences speech, causes increased dental caries (decay), and reduces artificial denture retention. Treatment includes reduction or elimination of agents causing dry mouth, or use of artificial saliva (available in pharmacies without a prescription) as a frequently applied lubricant for this annoying condition. Surgery is not required for dry mouth.

25. White Spots on Soft Tissue in Mouth (Fig. 12.20): Many conditions cause different types of white spots in the mouth, such as holding aspirin in the mouth, smoking, or eating hot foods. Some of these conditions are dangerous. If you have white spots in the mouth, you should definitely consult your dentist.

26. Hairy Tongue (Fig. 12.21): Black hairy tongue is not uncommon. It is not dangerous. Check with your dentist to find ways to reduce the collection of debris on your tongue.

27. Spots on Tongue (Fig. 12.22): Spots on the tongue, or "geographic tongue," is a com-

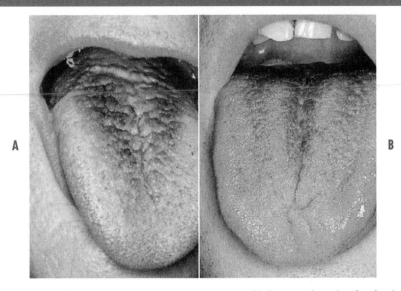

FIG. 12.21 **Hairy tongue is usually harmless.** (From Tyldesley WR: *Colour atlas of orofacial diseases*, ed 2, St Louis, 1991, Mosby [Wolfe]. Copyright 1991 by WR Tyldesley.)

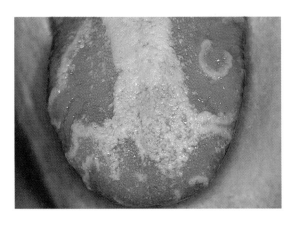

FIG. 12.22 **Spots on tongue (geographic tongue).** (From Regezi J, Sciubba J, Pogrel MA: *Atlas of oral and maxillofacial pathology*, Philadelphia, 2000, WB Saunders.)

monly occurring condition, in which the tongue looks like a map. It is not dangerous. Consult with your dentist to confirm the diagnosis.

WHAT YOUR ORAL AND MAXILLOFACIAL SURGEON OR GENERAL DENTIST CAN DO

Treatment Available

1. Biopsy

(Fig. 12.23). If a growth on the soft tissue (gum, lip, tongue, and so on) or hard tissue (bone) is suspicious, and a diagnosis cannot be determined by visual or radiographic (x-ray) observation, a small piece of tissue is removed surgically or with a stiff brush and examined under a microscope to aid in the diagnosis. This is a biopsy.

A. **Advantages:** The exact nature of the condition is confirmed microscopically.

B. **Disadvantages:** Some discomfort and cost are involved with a surgical biopsy.

C. **Risks:** There is a slight risk that the biopsy may stimulate further growth or systemic (body wide) distribution of the condition. If the unknown growth or other condition is small, a biopsy that removes all of the condition can be accomplished (excisional biopsy).

D. **Alternatives:** Removal of all suspect tissue is a good alternative. Waiting to see if the condition worsens is another alternative, but this is not usually suggested.

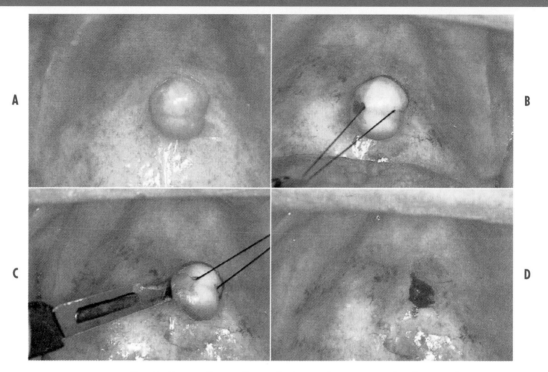

FIG. 12.23   A to D, Biopsy of an oral growth. (From McGowan DA: *An atlas of minor oral surgery: principles and practice,* ed 2, London, 1999, Martin Dunitz Ltd. Copyright 1999 by DA McGowan.)

E. **Cost:** A biopsy for oral conditions is relatively low in cost.

F. **Result of Nontreatment:** If a biopsy is indicated and is not accomplished, uncertainty about the surrounding area will continue until something happens to confirm the diagnosis.

2. Tooth Extraction

(Fig. 12.24). Various words are commonly used to describe tooth extractions: simple, surgical, partially bony, bony, and root removal. Extraction of an erupted tooth in a healthy individual is a relatively simple, nontraumatic event that heals well in a few days to a few weeks. Teeth that are functioning well or have the potential to do so with restorations (fillings, crowns [caps]), should not be extracted. Teeth that are highly diseased, are causing bone degeneration, and have a potential negative influence on overall body health should be removed.

Often, teeth are impacted (partially covered with soft tissue and/or bone) and may require extraction if the practitioner feels that they will not erupt adequately. Such impacted teeth usually have nothing wrong with them, except that they are in improper positions and cannot function. Leaving them in place can cause disease by development of cysts (growths in the bone) or deviation of other teeth. Some impacted teeth do not require extraction.

A. **Advantages:** Pain, discomfort, gum or bone disease, and improper tooth formation or positioning are eliminated.

B. **Disadvantages:** If the teeth to be extracted are functioning well, their extraction will reduce or eliminate proper function and impair the oral-facial appearance. Their extraction requires replacement. If teeth are impacted and serve no functional or appearance purposes, no disadvantages are involved.

C. **Risks:** Having teeth removed, implants placed, or other oral surgery ranges from a minor to major health risk. Simple extractions in healthy persons have few risks other than the normal, infrequent, expected risks of patient anes-

surgery has been accomplished and healing has occurred.

  A. **Advantages:** In some situations, surgical repositioning is the only procedure that can adequately establish a correct relationship between the jaws, desired appearance, or proper occlusion (bite). The procedures and healing take a relatively short time.

  B. **Disadvantages:** Some discomfort and significant costs are involved. However, patients usually inform practitioners that the discomfort is not as great as they had expected.

  C. **Risks:** Normal surgical risks are encountered (p. 92). It is also possible that the desired correction of the defect will not be complete and further surgery and/or orthodontic treatment (p. 107) will be needed.

  D. **Alternatives:** In a few situations, orthodontic therapy (p. 107), or extractions (p. 92) and aggressive fixed prosthodontic (p. 139) or removable prosthodontic (p. 155) therapy may satisfy the need. Talk to your practitioner to determine whether such alternatives are possible for you.

  E. **Cost:** You should expect to pay a significant fee for these services.

  F. **Result of Nontreatment:** The condition will continue to exist. In many situations the need for surgical repositioning is indicated primarily based on appearance; in these cases the original appearance defect will remain. Function may or may not continue to be negatively influenced.

8. Temporomandibular Joint Surgery, Arthroplasty

Conservative treatment of temporomandibular joint (TMJ) problems is almost always best (p. 77). However, in about 1% to 5% of TMJ or temporomandibular dysfunction (TMD) cases, surgery is indicated to correct the bone, ligaments, or muscle attachments related to the jaws. This condition is one for which several professional opinions are needed before treatment begins. The following practitioners known for their treatment of TMD should be consulted: prosthodontists (p. 15), periodontists (p. 14), some general dental practitioners, oral and maxillofacial surgeons (p. 11), and possibly an ear, nose, and throat specialist. The TMJ syndrome is complex, and you should not rush into treatment. At this time, TMJ surgery may be divided into two major categories: (1) conventional TMJ surgery requiring an incision, considerable rearrangement of TMJ parts, and a healing period; and (2) arthroplasty, in which a relatively innocuous skin penetration is made through which an arthroscope is inserted, allowing observation of the joint, minimal repairs and potential for inadvertent tissue destruction, and rapid healing.

  A. **Advantages:** TMJ surgery is rapid, effective, and can correct long-standing problems.

  B. **Disadvantages:** The surgery may not correct the condition. The procedure produces some discomfort and has significant cost.

  C. **Risks:** Normal surgical risks are encountered (p. 92).

  D. **Alternatives:** Waiting and tolerating signs and symptoms is the only alternative.

  E. **Cost:** TMJ surgery is difficult and has significant liability; the cost is moderate to high.

  F. **Result of Nontreatment:** Continued joint degeneration usually occurs, eventually requiring surgery.

9. Vestibuloplasty (Reforming Gum Tissues Over Jawbones to Create More Ridge) (Fig. 12.27).

After natural teeth have been out of the mouth for many years, the underlying bone and gums shrink considerably. The remaining bony ridge may not be sufficient to support a denture. One treatment for this condition is surgical repositioning of the soft tissue (gums) to provide more space on the front and back of the remaining bony ridge. The result is more ridge on which to place a denture. Sometimes the procedure is followed by placement of implants for further retention and support.

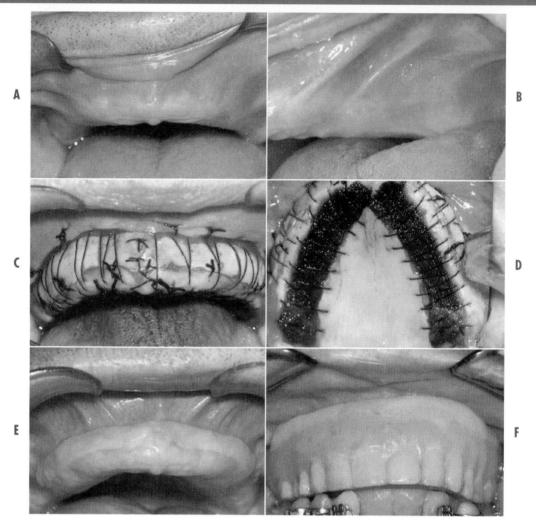

FIG. 12.27   A to F, Vestibuloplasty, showing operation beginning on top and ending with denture over newly formed ridge. (From Genco RJ, Goldman HM, Cohen W: *Contemporary periodontics*, St Louis, 1990, Mosby.)

A. **Advantages:** Presence of a larger, more stable ridge allows better support and function for the denture.
B. **Disadvantages:** There still may not be enough bone to hold a denture, and implants may be needed.
C. **Risks:** Normal surgical risks are encountered (p. 92).
D. **Alternatives:** Ridge augmentation (p. 94) or implants (p. 61) may be considered. Sometimes, all three—vestibuloplasty, ridge augmentation, and implants—may be needed.
E. **Cost:** You should expect moderate cost.
F. **Result of Nontreatment:** Continued and increasing inadequacy of denture support, function, and appearance should be expected.

SUMMARY

Surgery in the oral and maxillofacial regions is related to the elimination of pain and discomfort from diseased teeth, bones, and gums; removal of various growths; and changing the appearance and function of the jaws, teeth, and associated facial structures. Many local diseases of the oral-maxillofacial area are identifiable, and some local manifestations of overall body diseases are observed in this area. Your dentist and/or oral and maxillofacial surgeon can diagnose and treat these many conditions.

Orthodontics
Straightening Teeth

Most people have known someone who has needed to have teeth straightened. Malocclusion (poor bite and crooked teeth, **FIG. 13.1**) is one of the most common maladies in humans. There are many reasons why teeth do not develop into normal-appearing and functioning relationships. Among the most common is the well-known intermarrying of persons from different countries, races, or genetic backgrounds. Different persons have

different physical characteristics, and their children have random combinations of these features. The result is often large teeth in a small head or the reverse, and the appearance and function of the dentition is abnormal. It is doubtful that anyone has ever died because of crooked teeth, but the emotional distress caused by abnormal appearance of the smile does adversely affect personality. Also, the ability to eat can be negatively altered somewhat by teeth that do not occlude (bite) in a normal manner.

Assuming that the teeth of a person of any age seem to need orthodontic treatment, what is an appropriate way to have this treatment accomplished? Contrary to most other specialties in dentistry, orthodontic therapy is usually accomplished by orthodontists (p. 12) rather than general dentists. However, some general dentists and some pediatric dentists, with a special interest and some additional postdoctoral education, perform orthodontics. A logical sequence to follow is to consult a general dentist or dental specialist first to determine whether your teeth need orthodontic treatment. Usually, any dentist can give you an opinion as to whether orthodontics is indicated and can refer you to an orthodontist or other orthodontically oriented practitioner who can provide specific answers for you. In the event that the suggestions made during the orthodontic consultation are not clear, you should obtain a second opinion. Returning to the dentist who made the referral to discuss the orthodontic treatment plan is a good idea also.

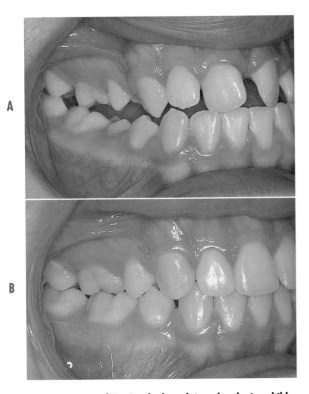

A

B

FIG. 13.1 **A and B,** Crooked teeth in a developing child are guided easily into a more normal position. (From Millett D, Welbury RR: *Colour guide orthodontics and paediatric dentistry,* 2000, Churchill Livingstone.)

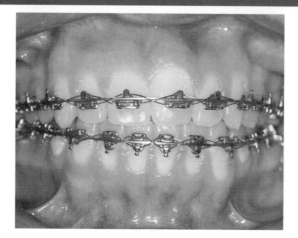

FIG. 13.2 **Fixed orthodontics—wires and brackets.**
(From Viazis AD: *Atlas of advanced orthodontics: a guide to clinical efficiency,* Philadelphia, 1998, WB Saunders.)

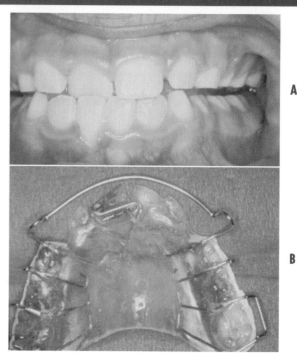

A

B

FIG. 13.3 **Removable orthodontic appliances. A,** Upper front teeth in proper bite relationship. **B,** Removable appliance to correct malocclusion. (From Cameron A, Widmer R: *Handbook of pediatric dentistry,* London, 1997, Mosby-Wolfe.)

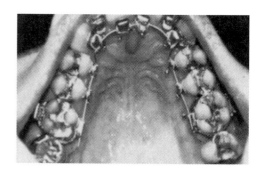

FIG. 13.4 **Invisible orthodontic appliances placed on tongue side of teeth.** (Courtesy Ormco Corporation.)

At what age should orthodontic therapy be accomplished? Many clinical situations require orthodontic therapy during childhood, and young children should be evaluated relative to the need for preventive orthodontics. Most orthodontic treatment is accomplished best and fastest during puberty. At that time, as the body is changing rapidly from adolescence to maturity, teeth move rapidly and easily in the supporting bone.

Can orthodontic therapy be accomplished in adulthood? Movement of teeth can and should (if needed) be accomplished at any time during life. If a person has the desire and can accept the time involved in orthodontic treatment, it should be considered. However, as the body matures and ages, the teeth are more difficult to move and also move more slowly than during youth. A few dental conditions, such as periodontal disease (p. 129) and some overall debilitating diseases, may preclude adult orthodontic therapy. Nevertheless, it is possible for most persons who need and want it.

Unlike most other oral treatment, orthodontics requires time for completion, ranging in youth from a few months to years, with a typical time of 1½ to 2 years. During this period patients wear various types of devices that move the teeth in the supporting bone by applying light force to achieve the desired position. Orthodontic appliances range from fixed brackets or bands and wires on the teeth **(FIG. 13.2)** to removable appliances **(FIG. 13.3),** or combinations of both. Some orthodontic therapy can be accomplished by nearly invisible appliances, so-called lingual (tongue side of teeth) appliances **(FIG. 13.4).** Although you can certainly express an opinion about your preference for the type of orthodontic appliance used for you, the practitioner accomplishing the therapy should be allowed to select the type most appropriate for your needs.

Is there discomfort during orthodontic therapy? Yes, teeth are moved through supporting bone by placing slight, well-directed forces on the part of the tooth that is observable in the mouth (the crown). As an orthodontic appliance on the tooth places force on the bone, the bone on the pressure side of the tooth degenerates, and the bone on the other side of the tooth, where there is no pressure, fills bone into the space created. If this procedure is performed too rapidly, discomfort and damage can occur. Your orthodontist certainly knows the amount of force to apply to teeth. There is usually minor discomfort during orthodontic therapy, especially right after the appliances have been tightened and for a short time thereafter.

Can all crooked teeth or malalignment of jaws be corrected by orthodontics? No, some situations require surgical correction (p. 95). The need for combined surgery and orthodontic therapy does not occur frequently, and your orthodontist will suggest this therapy if it appears to be the best choice. If orthognathic surgery is suggested, a second professional opinion is usually advisable.

Orthodontic therapy has improved the appearance of millions of people, allowing them to chew more thoroughly, and, most importantly, feel better about themselves. A person who does not feel normal in appearance often withdraws from social interaction. Crooked or otherwise unsightly teeth and an unpleasant smile can negatively influence personality and self-esteem.

WHAT YOU SEE OR FEEL

Conditions, Signs, and Symptoms Related to Orthodontic Treatment

1. Front and/or Back Teeth Crooked

(FIG. 13.5). Almost everybody has some malalignment of teeth, but when the teeth appear to be markedly different from what is considered normal, the person is often bothered by his or her appearance. There is an extreme variation in the crookedness of teeth, ranging from slightly malpositioned to the point that correction of the appearance looks nearly

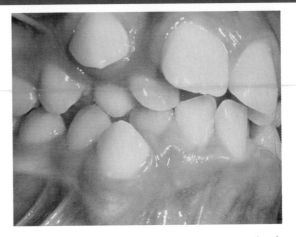

FIG. 13.5   Malalignment of teeth. (From Viazis AD: *Atlas of advanced orthodontics: a guide to clinical efficiency*, Philadelphia, 1998, WB Saunders.)

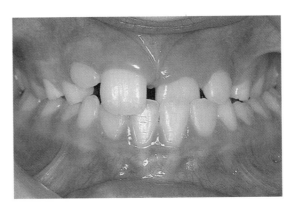

FIG. 13.6   Malocclusion of teeth. Jaws close into crossbite, but correctly aligned jaw relationship causes open bite. (From Millett D, Welbury RR: *Colour guide orthodontics and paediatric dentistry*, 2000, Churchill Livingstone.)

hopeless to an observer. Most crooked teeth can be improved significantly by orthodontic therapy (p. 107). Occasionally the teeth are so large or small for the size of the jaws that surgery (p. 95) may be necessary to correct this tooth-jaw discrepancy after or during orthodontic therapy.

2. Front or Back Teeth Don't Come Together Correctly When Jaws are Closed (Malocclusion)

(FIG. 13.6). Teeth usually erupt until they touch opposing teeth on the other jaw. The most frequently encountered reason that teeth do not occlude (come together) is that some object, such as the tongue, is routinely placed between them. One variation of this habit is a

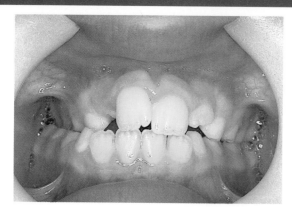

FIG. 13.7 **Crossbite on patient's right side.** (From Millett D, Welbury RR: *Colour guide orthodontics and paediatric dentistry*, 2000, Churchill Livingstone.)

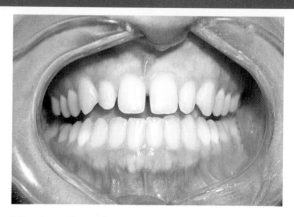

FIG. 13.8 **Spaces between teeth can be solved by orthodontic treatment, bonding, or crowns (caps).**

"tongue thrust," in which the patient places the tongue between the teeth during swallowing. You can check for the condition easily by placing a small amount of water in the mouth and parting the lips slightly while swallowing to observe the tongue. If a tongue thrust is present, the tongue will move forcefully forward while the water is being swallowed. Other situations that cause teeth to remain apart during jaw closure include thumb or finger sucking, pipe smoking, habitual tongue biting or sucking, and many other conditions. Your dentist or orthodontist can usually tell you what has caused the teeth to remain apart. Orthodontic therapy (p. 107) along with correcting the habit that caused the open bite usually corrects the condition, but surgery may be necessary if the condition is extreme.

3. Some or All Teeth Are in a Crossbite Condition When Jaws Close (Upper Teeth Close Behind Lower Teeth)

(FIG. 13.7). Crossbites can usually be corrected by routine orthodontic therapy (p. 107), and only infrequently is surgery (p. 95) required. Occasionally a crossbite can be treated by placing crowns (caps).

4. Spaces Between Teeth

(FIG. 13.8). Spaces between teeth range from minor ones that collect objectionable pieces of food to large, unsightly spaces that could nearly accommodate another tooth. As with most situations for which orthodontics is an elective

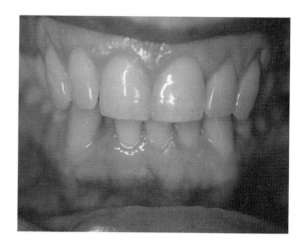

FIG. 13.9 **Deviated midline.** (From Viazis AD: *Atlas of advanced orthodontics: a guide to clinical efficiency*, Philadelphia, 1998, WB Saunders.)

therapy, the spaces do not cause any damage except to the appearance. If the spaces are large, orthodontic therapy is necessary (p. 107), but if they are small, patients may prefer the faster results of bonding (filling spaces with small additions of plastic to the teeth, p. 54) or crowns (caps) (p. 146). In severe cases, extremely large spaces may allow only removal of teeth and placement of a partial or complete denture (p. 162).

5. Midline of Teeth Is Obviously Left or Right of the Midline of the Face When Smiling

(FIG. 13.9). Malpositioning of the teeth in the jaw(s) can cause the midline to be nonsymmetrical with the rest of the face. Almost all people have some deviation of the nose to one

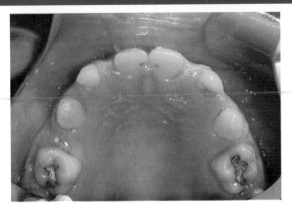

FIG. 13.10   **Several permanent teeth failed to develop in this patient.**

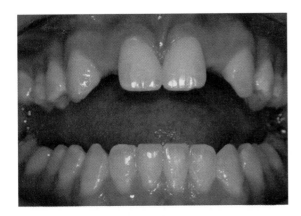

FIG. 13.11   **Missing upper lateral incisors requiring either orthodontic treatment or tooth replacement with implants and crowns (caps), fixed prostheses (bridges), or other therapy.**

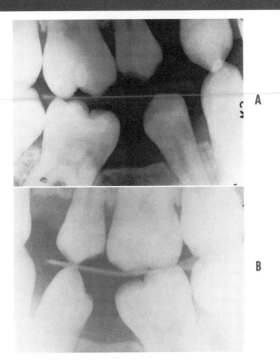

FIG. 13.12   **A and B, Missing lower premolars caused tipping of adjacent teeth and the need for orthodontic treatment.** (From Proffit WR: *Contemporary orthodontics,* ed 2, St Louis, 1993, Mosby.)

side or the other, and this condition can be misleading when considering the correct location of the midline. However, to be symmetrical, the midline of the teeth should appear to be halfway between the centers of the pupils of the eyes when the person is looking straight ahead. This placement of teeth has no significance physiologically, but extreme variation can cause a significant defect in appearance. Usually, orthodontic therapy (p. 107) can correct the condition, but occasionally, surgery must be a part of the treatment plan also (p. 95).

6. Spaces Where Some Teeth Did Not Develop

(FIG. 13.10). Many people have missing teeth because the teeth did not develop or erupt. These conditions are usually genetic and are passed from parents to children. The most

commonly missing teeth are upper lateral incisors **(FIG. 13.11)** or lower premolars **(FIG. 13.12).** Carefully positioned radiographs (x-rays) must be made to determine if the apparently missing teeth are in fact missing. Occasionally, teeth are present under the bone and gums and have not erupted into the mouth because other teeth block them. These teeth can be surgically stimulated to erupt, and they may or may not need orthodontic therapy for assisted eruption.

Missing teeth can be replaced with fixed prostheses (p. 149), implants followed by crowns (caps) (p. 72), or removable prostheses (p. 70), or by moving surrounding teeth orthodontically to fill the spaces (p. 107). It seems most logical to move natural teeth into the spaces orthodontically, thereby eliminating the need to make artificial replacements.

7. Teeth Slant Downhill to the Right or Left When Smiling

(FIG. 13.13). Forces present during facial development, genetic disorders, or peculiar habits such as thumb sucking can cause teeth to be out of line with the normally expected tooth

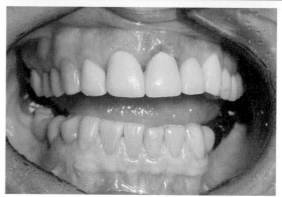

FIG. 13.13 **Downhill slant of lower teeth.**

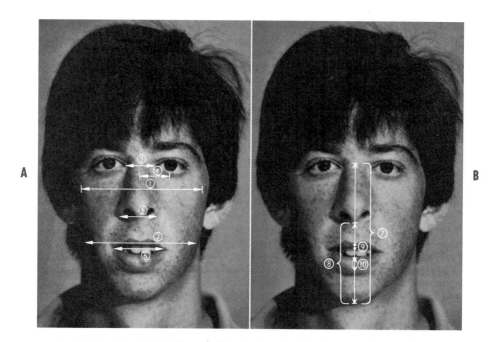

FIG. 13.14 **A and B,** Smiling parallels the imaginary line between the pupils. (From Proffit WR, Fields HW Jr: *Contemporary orthodontics,* ed 3, St Louis, 2000, Mosby.)

alignment. Usually the orientation of the front teeth when smiling is parallel to an imaginary line drawn between the pupils of the eyes **(FIG. 13.14).** Any notable deviation from that relationship often produces an objectionable abnormal appearance.

After a dentist or dental specialist has ruled out any reasons for continued development of this problem, correction of the unsightly appearance can be accomplished in the following ways:

A. Simple incisal recontouring (changing the length or other contour of the teeth by carefully grinding and smoothing them) (p. 54)

B. Orthodontic movement of the teeth (p. 107)

C. Placement of veneers (p. 55)

D. Placement of crowns (caps) (p. 146)

E. In extreme cases, surgery to reposition the teeth and surrounding bone (p. 95)

Orthodontic treatment or recontouring teeth are the most preferred and conservative methods.

8. Gums Show Too Much When Smiling

(FIG. 13.15). Numerous conditions make the gums dominate the smile. Among these are medications given for various physical conditions that stimulate the gums to overgrow; lips that lift high during smiling, exposing display of the gums; a maxilla (upper jaw) that is larger than normal; or lack of the normal gum shrinkage that usually occurs throughout ado-

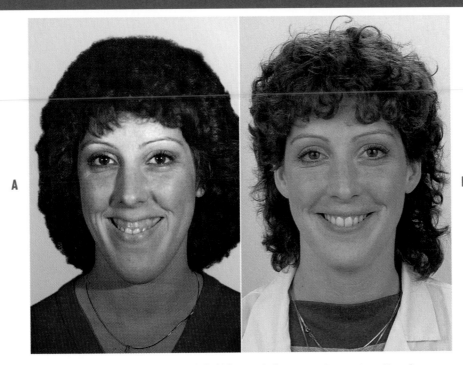

FIG. 13.15   A and B, Gummy smile before and after corrective surgery. (From Sarver DM: *Esthetic orthodontics and orthognathic surgery,* St Louis, 1998, Mosby.)

lescence and early adulthood. Some of the treatments for gums that show too much during smiling are:

  A. Surgery to remove some of the gum tissue from the teeth, thereby exposing more tooth structure (p. 135)
  B. Orthodontic treatment to move the teeth back up into the gums and bone (p. 107), followed by surgery to remove excess gums (p. 135)
  C. Orthognathic surgery to move the entire upper jaw upward, thereby removing the excess gum tissue displayed (p. 95)

9. Natural Teeth Do Not Show When Smiling

Various conditions cause a lack of display of natural teeth when smiling. Among them are excessive wear of natural teeth (bruxism or clenching, p. 76) to the degree that they do not show; inadequate growth of the maxilla (upper jaw), thus keeping the upper teeth hidden under the lip; or a naturally long lip. Correction of this lack of tooth display during smiling can be accomplished by the following treatments:

  A. Orthognathic surgery to build up the upper jaw (maxilla) (p. 95)
  B. Crowns (caps) (p. 146) or other prostheses to build up the teeth

  C. Orthodontic therapy to pull the upper teeth and the bone down further, thereby displaying them during smiling (p. 107)

10. Upper Teeth Too Far Backward, With Upper Jaw Appearing Underdeveloped

(FIG. 13.16). This condition may be either an underdeveloped upper jaw or an overdeveloped lower jaw. True underdevelopment of the upper jaw (retrognathia) is usually treated best by orthodontic movement of teeth to the preferred position in the dental bone (alveolus), followed by movement of the entire jaw by orthognathic surgery (p. 95).

11. Lower Teeth Too Far Forward

(FIG. 13.17). Often called *lantern jaw,* this condition is usually treated best with surgery (p. 95) to move the jaw backward and correct the jaw relationship. Orthodontic therapy (p. 107) may be required before and/or after the surgery to place the teeth in correct position.

12. Baby (Primary) Teeth Retained in Place, Permanent Teeth Unerupted

(FIG. 13.18). Retained primary teeth can serve well for years, or their roots can resorb (degenerate) without stimulation, requiring ex-

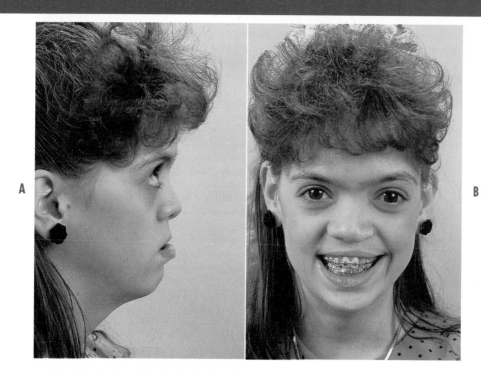

FIG. 13.16　A and B, Underdeveloped upper jaw; patient undergoing orthodontic therapy. (From Sarver DM: *Esthetic orthodontics and orthognathic surgery,* St Louis, 1998, Mosby.)

FIG. 13.17　Lower teeth too far forward. (From Millett D, Welbury RR: *Colour guide orthodontics and paediatric dentistry,* 2000, Churchill Livingstone.)

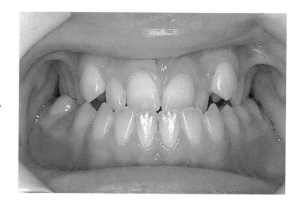

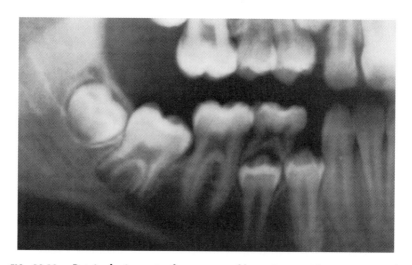

FIG. 13.18　Retained primary teeth on upper and lower jaws, with permanent teeth unable to erupt properly. (From Proffit WR, Fields HW Jr: *Contemporary orthodontics,* ed 3, St Louis, 2000, Mosby.)

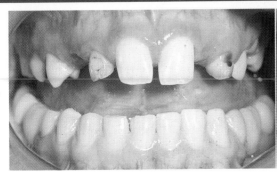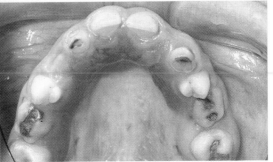

A   **B**

FIG. 13.19   **A and B,** Crooked primary (baby) teeth.

traction. When strong primary teeth remain in place without degenerate roots, they should be left until the roots degenerate. If root resorption (degeneration) has occurred, they should be removed, followed by orthodontic movement (p. 107) of the teeth to fill the space, or an implant followed by a crown (cap) (p. 146), a fixed prosthesis (bridge) (p. 149), or a removable prosthesis (p. 162). If permanent teeth are unable to erupt because primary (baby) teeth remain in position, the primary teeth should be extracted, allowing room for the permanent teeth to erupt.

13. Baby Teeth (Primary Teeth) Crooked

(FIG. 13.19). Orthodontic tooth movement can be accomplished on primary teeth, but unless an extreme condition is present, orthodontic therapy usually is delayed until the permanent teeth are in place. Sometimes, primary and permanent teeth in the mouth at the same time (mixed dentition) can be moved slightly with minor orthodontic therapy, called *interceptive orthodontics* (p. 111), to prevent the occurrence of a more severe orthodontic need later.

WHAT YOUR ORTHODONTIST, PEDIATRIC DENTIST, OR GENERAL DENTIST CAN DO

Treatment Available

Teeth may be moved in numerous ways, and each method has advocates and critics. In fact, the best method to accomplish orthodontic treatment is among the most controversial subjects in dentistry. Consumers of orthodontic services should be concerned only that they receive safe tooth movement in a reasonable time that accomplishes the desired result: straight teeth and/or a correct bite.

1. Orthodontic Treatment

(FIG. 13.20). Some of the more popular ways to accomplish orthodontic movement of teeth include:

- **Metal Bands and Wires Placed on Teeth** (FIG. 13.21). Metal bands and wires allow slight forces to be placed accurately on the part of the tooth that is visible above the gums (the crown). These forces are applied by wires and/or elastics, and the teeth move to the desired positions. Although metal banding is one of the oldest and best methods to move teeth orthodontically, metal bands are unsightly, and they require that a slight space is developed between the teeth for adequate placement of the bands. These spaces are closed later.

- **Bonded Plastic or Ceramic Brackets and Wires Placed on Teeth** (FIG. 13.22). These mechanisms are a newer concept to apply orthodontic force. These brackets are applied by acid etching the teeth similar to bonding (p. 54), placing plastic cement on the roughened surface, and cementing the bracket into place. Brackets are better in appearance than metal bands, but their removal often leaves a considerable amount of debris that must be removed carefully after the orthodontic therapy is concluded.

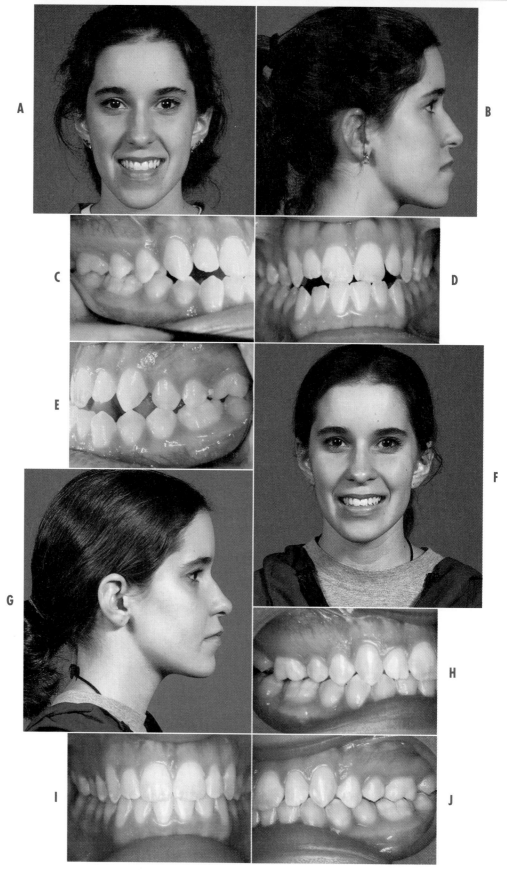

FIG. 13.20 **A to E,** Before orthodontic treatment. **F to J,** After orthodontic treatment. (From Proffit WR, Fields HW Jr: *Contemporary orthodontics,* ed 3, St Louis, 2000, Mosby.)

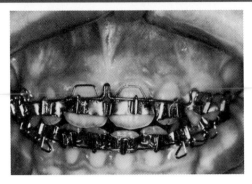

FIG. 13.21   Metal bands and wires. (From Proffit WR, Fields HW Jr: *Contemporary orthodontics,* ed 3, St Louis, 2000, Mosby.)

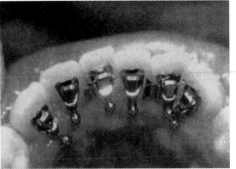

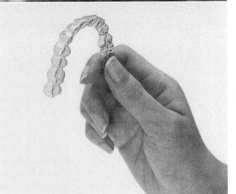

FIG. 13.23   A, Invisible brackets placed on tongue side of teeth. **B,** The "Aligner" by Invisalign. (**A** Courtesy Ormco Corporation. **B** Courtesy Align Technology Inc, Santa Clara, Calif.)

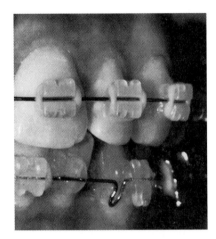

FIG. 13.22   Ceramic brackets. (From Proffit WR, Fields HW Jr: *Contemporary orthodontics,* ed 3, St Louis, 2000, Mosby.)

- **Invisible Brackets (FIG. 13.23).** Invisible bracket mechanisms may sometimes be placed on surfaces of the teeth adjacent to the tongue (Fig. 13.23, *A*) to provide forces to the teeth without the unsightly appearance of metal bands or plastic brackets. Only some tooth-movement needs may be adapted to this type of orthodontic device, but if your vocation or other reasons demand that you do not show bands or brackets during tooth movement, you should ask your practitioner about this type of service.

    An orthodontic treatment that does not require metal brackets or wires is available (FIG. 13.23, *B*). This therapy can treat up to 80% of people over the age of 15 who qualify for braces. The treatment uses three-dimensional computer imaging technology to create a series of clear, custom-made, removable aligners.

Each set of aligners is worn for about 2 weeks, gradually moving a patient's teeth to the prescribed position.

- **Removable Orthodontic Appliances (FIG. 13.24).** Some orthodontic needs are satisfied with removable devices. Others are better completed with fixed bands or brackets, and some require use of both fixed and removable devices. After completing orthodontic treatment, most patients need to wear a removable appliance called a retainer or space maintainer while the new positioning of teeth produced by the orthodontic therapy matures in the supportive bone.

A. **Advantages of Orthodontic Therapy:** Improvement in appearance and the resulting boost in self-acceptance cannot be measured but is highly important. Self-esteem is at its lowest during the adolescent years, and improvement in appearance at that time can significantly change the overall life of the orthodontic patient. Chewing function sometimes improves after treatment, but the significance of this change is not usually the

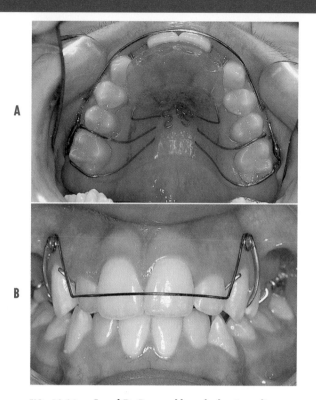

FIG. 13.24 **A and B,** Removable orthodontic appliances. (From Millett D, Welbury RR: *Colour guide orthodontics and paediatric dentistry,* 2000, Churchill Livingstone.)

main reason for orthodontic service. Stabilization of the occlusion (bite) by having maximum opposing tooth contact may improve the health of the jaw joints, but even this characteristic is debated strongly among those in various segments of the dental profession. It seems that the major reasons for orthodontic therapy are improving the appearance of the smile and upgrading the ability of the teeth to chew food well. Extremely crooked teeth or malaligned jaws may have more major physiological reasons.

B. **Disadvantages:** Time is required for orthodontic tooth movement, and some discomfort is experienced. The appearance of the smile is usually cluttered with brackets, bands, wires, elastics, or other devices for many months, and the cost of the therapy is significant. It is difficult to clean properly around teeth with orthodontic appliances on them.

C. **Risks:** When accomplished in a careful manner on a healthy person, very few risks occur during orthodontic therapy. However, even when every precaution is taken, a few risks must be considered. It is difficult to clean teeth with fixed orthodontic appliances on them, and removable orthodontic devices hold food and debris against the teeth. These unclean conditions are conducive to dental caries (decay), and every precaution must be taken to avoid increased decay during orthodontic therapy (p. 107). Use of topically applied preventive fluorides, rinses, fluoride toothpastes, and mechanical toothbrushes are encouraged during this time.

Occasionally, tooth movement can cause a tooth pulp (nerve) (p. 37) to die, requiring endodontic (root canal) therapy for that tooth (p. 40).

Infrequently, tooth movement stimulates resorption (degeneration) of a part of the root of the tooth, weakening the support of the tooth and potentially causing the need for endodontics (root canal therapy).

D. **Alternatives:** If all or most of the teeth in the mouth are malpositioned, good alternatives are not available, other than doing nothing and living with the situation. If only a few front teeth are involved, crowns (caps) (p. 146) or veneers (small pieces of plastic or porcelain to change the shape of teeth) (p. 55) can be placed to recontour the teeth into a normal-appearing relationship. If the front teeth are too crooked and malpositioned to be straightened by just a few crowns (caps) or veneers, a few teeth may be removed (p. 92) and a fixed prosthesis (fixed bridge) (p. 149) or removable prosthesis (removable partial denture) (p. 162) can be placed **(FIG. 13.25)** to satisfy appearance needs. Removal of teeth and replacement with a prosthesis is usually faster than orthodontic treatment, but it may cost as much as or more than orthodontic tooth movement.

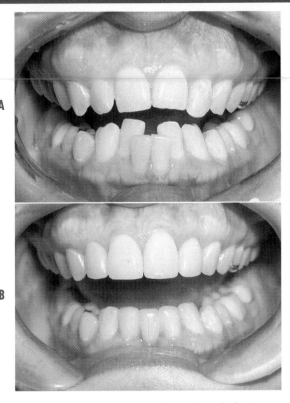

FIG. 13.25   **A** and **B,** An alternative for orthodontic treatment: Two lower teeth were removed and a fixed prosthesis placed on the lower arch. The upper four front teeth received veneers to lengthen them.

E. **Cost:** Although the cost of having all of the teeth moved to the most acceptable places seems high, it can be compared with many other popular consumer items, such as a large television, that have little or no long-term positive value for the family. Orthodontic treatment is a bargain when based on the expertise required of the practitioner and clinical auxiliary personnel, the many visits necessary during therapy, and the good that it does for the patient.

F. **Result of Nontreatment:** The major result of leaving crooked, malpositioned, unsightly teeth as they are is the continuation of diminished self-esteem caused by the condition. The negative psychological influence caused by this facial defect is not known, but it is probably significant over a lifetime. Some less significant influences in chewing function will continue and potentially increase without orthodontic therapy.

2. Interceptive Orthodontics

(FIG. 13.26). As a child grows and matures, many indications are apparent to dentists that the child's teeth may not develop into normal positioning relationships. Practitioners with an orientation toward this concept may warn parents of the potential need for orthodontic therapy, and they may suggest some type of minor orthodontic therapy during an early developmental time in the child's life.

A. **Advantages:** Minor preventive orthodontic procedures can often prevent major problems from developing later. Discomfort is reduced, and time and money are often saved.

B. **Disadvantages:** Cost to the family and inconvenience are present early in the child's life. Occasionally the result of the interceptive procedure cannot be predicted totally before it is accomplished.

C. **Risks:** The risks are the same as for orthodontic therapy (p. 107), but usually to a lesser degree.

D. **Alternatives:** Waiting to see if the child's dentition develops normally without orthodontic therapy is an alternative, but indicators of the development of orthodontic problems are quite clear, and waiting is not an alternative without predictable risk.

E. **Cost:** The costs are lower for interceptive procedures than for full orthodontic therapy because interceptive therapy is usually much less comprehensive. Also, many general dentists and most pediatric dentists offer this therapy, and interceptive orthodontics prevents the challenge of getting involved with an orthodontic practitioner in a new location.

F. **Result of Nontreatment:** If the practitioner suggesting interceptive orthodontics has made the correct diagnosis, the result of nontreatment is clear: The patient will eventually need full orthodontic therapy, which will usually cost more than the interceptive care. Also,

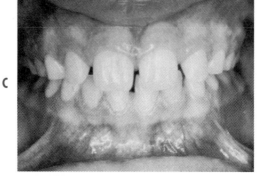

FIG. 13.26   A to C, Interceptive orthodontics at an early age often prevents major orthodontic treatment later. (From McDonald RE, Avery DR: *Dentistry for the child and adolescent,* ed 7, St Louis, 2000, Mosby.)

the treatment could be significantly more difficult because the interceptive work was not done.

SUMMARY

Orthodontics is usually among the most elective areas of oral therapy. However, when considering the significant effect on personality development that a beautiful smile with normally aligned teeth can have, and the increased self-esteem that this health service develops, it becomes less elective. Orthodontic therapy, usually delivered by orthodontic specialists, is readily available at moderate cost and without many risks or complications. It should be accomplished when necessary to improve the appearance of the smile and the function of the chewing mechanism, as well as to improve patient self-acceptance.

CHAPTER 14

Pediatric Dentistry
Dentistry for Children

Pediatric dentistry has evolved because of the special psychological challenges of children and the occasional peculiar clinical conditions that are present in children. Most dentistry performed for children is rendered by general dentists, but many situations are treated best by a pediatric dentist (children's specialist). Your general dentist can advise you on whether your child should see a pediatric dentist, or you may prefer to find a pediatric dentist just because most of them have practices that are oriented completely toward the special needs of children.

Many oral conditions of children are not so different from those conditions of adults, and you will be referred to other parts of this book for details on those conditions. However, continuing growth of the body, and eruption and eventual loss of the primary (baby) teeth during childhood present some special challenges. Also, a major problem observed in some children is a tremendous fear of health practitioners, developed by a previous bad experience or by unknowing family or friends. These psychological challenges usually require more special effort for the practitioner than do the clinical challenges.

Initial childhood dental experiences often set children's lifelong attitudes toward dentistry. Preventive concepts initiated and maintained for children relate directly to their long-term oral health. The level of a child's oral hygiene relates to the retention of the natural teeth for life or their premature loss. It is highly important that a proper introduction to dentistry be made for children as early as possible (age 6 to 12 months), and that close observation and/or therapy be continued every 6 months for life.

This chapter discusses only those conditions and treatments that are specific to children (from birth to teens), because the other conditions, which occur in both adults and children, are covered elsewhere in this book and are referenced.

WHAT YOU SEE OR FEEL

Conditions, Signs, or Symptoms Related to Pediatric Dentistry

1. Holes in Primary (Baby) Teeth, Often Discolored (Black, Gray, Brown, Yellow, Chalky) (FIG. 14.1). Dental caries (decay) in children is similar to adult tooth decay. However, in children the disease may be in the primary (baby) teeth. These smaller teeth do not have a great amount of enamel on them, and the decay process can progress rapidly. When decay is

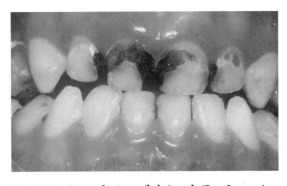

FIG. 14.1 **Decayed primary (baby) teeth.** (From Cameron A, Widmer R: *Handbook of pediatric dentistry*, London, 1997, Mosby-Wolfe.)

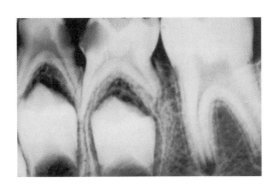

FIG. 14.2 **Tooth decay with pulp (nerve) involvement. Note dark holes in teeth.** (From McDonald RE, Avery DR: *Dentistry for the child and adolescent*, ed 7, St Louis, 2000, Mosby.)

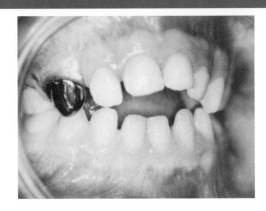

FIG. 14.5 **Stainless steel crowns (caps) are unpleasant in appearance, but they serve well.** (From McDonald RE, Avery DR: *Dentistry for the child and adolescent*, ed 7, St Louis, 2000, Mosby.)

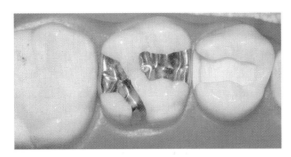

FIG. 14.3 **Amalgam restorations (fillings) on primary (baby) teeth. Note trimmed tooth on the right, ready for restoration.**

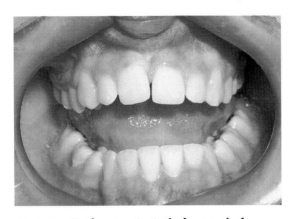

FIG. 14.4 **Tooth restoration in the front teeth of an adolescent. You can't tell which teeth are restored.**

found at an early stage, typical fillings can be placed in the primary teeth with reasonable assurance of years of longevity. When dental caries has progressed to involve the dental pulp (nerve) **(FIG. 14.2)**, either a root canal can be done on a permanent tooth (p. 40), or a pulpotomy (p. 124) can be done on a primary tooth.

If the dental carious lesion is large and/or the pulp (nerve) is exposed, it is likely that in the back teeth a stainless steel crown (cap), or in the front teeth a tooth-colored crown (cap) will be required to strengthen primary teeth. Alternatives include the following:

A. Silver amalgam restorations (fillings) **(FIG. 14.3**, p. 170)

B. Tooth-colored restorations **(FIG. 14.4**, p. 173)

C. Stainless steel crowns (caps) **(FIG. 14.5**, p. 125)

D. Tooth-colored crowns (caps) **(FIG. 14.6**, p. 146)

E. Removing the primary (baby) tooth (p. 126) and placing a space maintainer **(FIG. 14.7**, p. 128)

F. Pulpotomy (p. 124) and crown (cap) (p. 146)

2. Permanent Tooth Won't Erupt (Come into Mouth)

(FIG. 14.8). After the primary teeth exfoliate (come out), the permanent teeth are usually present within a few days or weeks. However, permanent teeth occasionally are slow to come in for several reasons: premature loss of primary teeth stimulated by trauma; abnormal positioning of permanent or primary teeth, not allowing permanent teeth to erupt **(FIG. 14.9)**; and lack of formation and presence of permanent teeth. Usually it is of little concern when teeth are slow to erupt, but occasionally there is a problem. If you have any

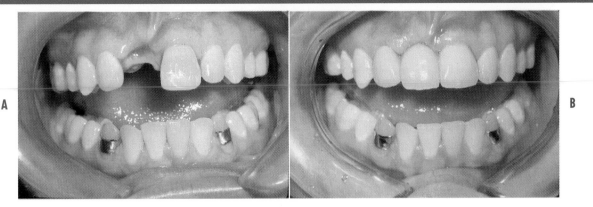

FIG. 14.6   **A** and **B,** Tooth-colored crowns (caps) are nearly undetectable from natural teeth. This teenager has one missing tooth replaced with a fixed prosthesis (bridge) connected to one tooth on each side of the space.

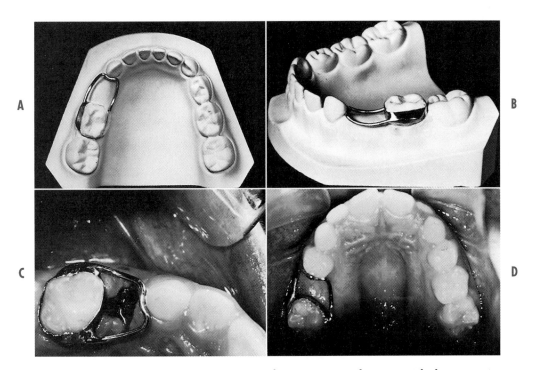

FIG. 14.7   **A to D,** Space maintainers are of various types and are essential when back teeth are lost. (From Proffit WR, Fields HW Jr: *Contemporary orthodontics,* ed 3, St Louis, 2000, Mosby.)

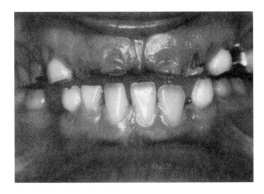

FIG. 14.8   **Unerupted teeth.** (From Koch G et al: *Pedodontics: a clinical approach,* Copenhagen, 1991, Munksgaard.)

Pediatric Dentistry

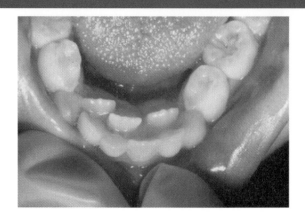

FIG. 14.9   **Malpositioned primary (baby) teeth can retard the eruption of permanent teeth. Note four primary upper teeth preventing proper eruption of permanent teeth.** (From Cameron A, Widmer R: *Handbook of pediatric dentistry,* London, 1997, Mosby-Wolfe.)

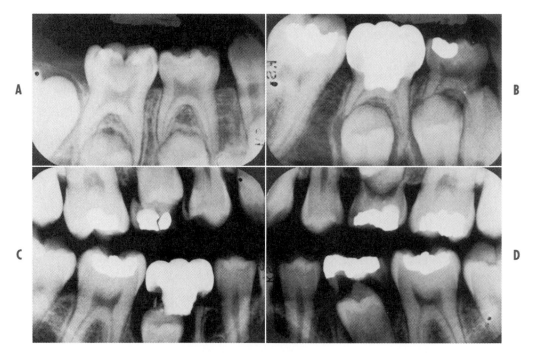

FIG. 14.10   **A to D,** Radiographs of unerupted teeth show permanent teeth held in unerupted state by primary (baby) teeth retained too long. (From McDonald RE, Avery DR: *Dentistry for the child and adolescent,* ed 7, St Louis, 2000, Mosby.)

question, you should consult a professional. Alternatives include the following:

A. Wait a longer time for the tooth eruption.

B. Obtain a radiograph (x-ray) to see if any problem is present and continue to wait for eruption **(FIG. 14.10).**

C. Assisted eruption: the dentist encourages the tooth to erupt by making a channel in the overlying gum tissue and/or underlying bone.

D. Assisted eruption with orthodontics: the dentist encourages the tooth to erupt by making a channel in the gum tissue and bone and attaching a device to the nonerupted tooth to help bring it slowly into place **(FIG. 14.11).**

3. Dark-Colored Primary Tooth

(FIG. 14.12). Children often suffer an accidental blow to a primary tooth. Sometimes the parent may not even know it happened. Later the tooth turns dark. Usually the tooth pulp (nerve) **(FIG. 14.13)** has been injured, and the dark coloration is caused by degenerative pigments in the blood supply to the nerve inside the tooth. This condition may

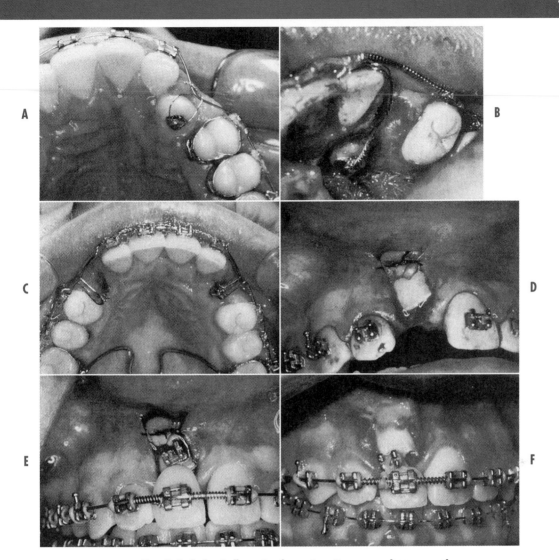

FIG. 14.11   **A** to **F,** Orthodontically assisted eruption. From top to bottom are the various stages in assisted eruption of teeth, a slow but successful treatment. (From Proffit WR, Fields HW Jr: *Contemporary orthodontics,* ed 2, St Louis, 1993, Mosby.)

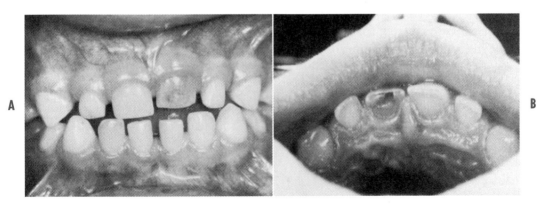

FIG. 14.12   **A** and **B,** Dark primary (baby) tooth caused by trauma. (From McDonald RE, Avery DR: *Dentistry for the child and adolescent,* ed 7, St Louis, 2000, Mosby.)

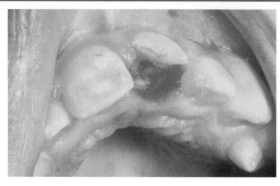

FIG. 14.13 **The pulp (nerve) of a child's tooth has been exposed by trauma, requiring pulp capping and a filling (restoration).** (From Cameron A, Widmer R: *Handbook of pediatric dentistry,* London, 1997, Mosby-Wolfe.)

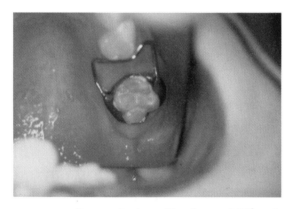

FIG. 14.14 **Space maintainers.** (From Cameron A, Widmer R: *Handbook of pediatric dentistry,* London, 1997, Mosby-Wolfe.)

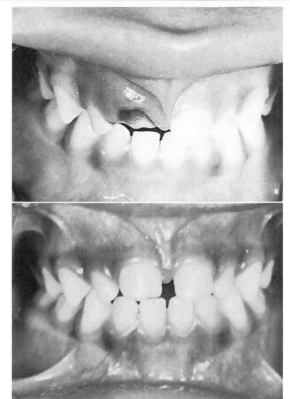

FIG. 14.15 **A, The primary tooth forced into gum. B, Tooth re-erupted during a period of 8 months.** (From McDonald RE, Avery DR: *Dentistry for the child and adolescent,* ed 7, St Louis, 2000, Mosby.)

or may not be painful. Alternatives include the following:

A. If the tooth is not painful, leave it in place with its dark color unchanged.
B. Remove a part or all of the nerve of the tooth (pulpotomy or pulpectomy), and bleach the tooth back to a near-normal color.
C. Remove the tooth (p. 126) and place a space maintainer **(FIG. 14.14)**, (p. 128).

4. Primary or Permanent Tooth Accidentally Forced into Gum Tissue and Bone

(FIG. 14.15). A primary or permanent tooth may be accidentally pushed forcefully into the underlying bone and soft tissue. If the child is only a few years old, there may be a problem with the underlying partially developed permanent tooth; the primary tooth could injure the developing tooth bud of the permanent tooth. However, if the child is older, and depending on which tooth is involved, the underlying permanent tooth may not be damaged. Damage to an underlying permanent tooth cannot be determined completely until the suspect tooth erupts later. If the primary tooth is severely fractured under the gum, it may need to be removed. If the tooth is a permanent one, the damage is usually related only to the tooth receiving the blow. Alternatives include the following:

A. Leave the tooth intruded and let it work back into its normal position over time. Teeth with only minor displacement will adapt to this conservative option.
B. Have your dentist gently move the tooth manually to place it back in its

A   B   C

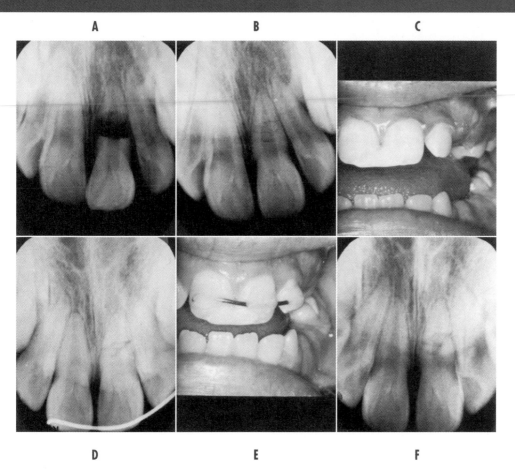

D   E   F

FIG. 14.16   A to F, Tooth stabilization from upper left to lower right; fractured tooth was stabilized with plastic and wire until healing took place, after which wire and plastic were removed. (From McDonald RE, Avery DR: *Dentistry for the child and adolescent*, ed 7, St Louis, 2000, Mosby.)

original position. The dentist may have to stabilize the tooth **(FIG. 14.16)** to allow it to heal back into the correct location.

C. Have the tooth removed if it is severely fractured below the bone or if its root is fractured into two or more loose pieces in the bone. If the tooth is removed, a space maintainer is usually needed (see Fig. 14.14), (p. 128).

5. Infant or Young Child With Multiple Decayed Teeth, Especially in Front of Mouth

(FIG. 14.17). This condition is often called the *bottle mouth syndrome* or *baby bottle syndrome.* It involves allowing the child to suck a bottle of any sugar-containing substance for hours at a time. Teeth are usually decayed slightly to severely and require selection of

one of the alternatives described previously in the first section "Holes in Primary Teeth" (p. 113).

6. Upper and Lower Front Teeth Do Not Come Together (Open Bite)

(FIG. 14.18). Habits such as thumb or finger sucking, or habitually holding some object between the teeth, will not allow the teeth to come together in the area of the object being sucked. Placing the tongue between the teeth when swallowing will commonly cause an open bite in the front of the mouth. This tongue thrust condition is often not known by the child or parent until they are informed. Alternatives include the following:

A. Leave the condition as it is and accept the open bite.

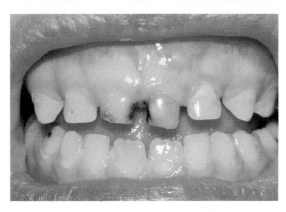

FIG. 14.17   Multiple decayed teeth caused by sucking bottle filled with sugar-containing juice (bottle mouth syndrome or baby bottle syndrome).

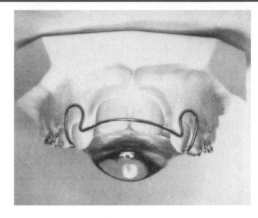

FIG. 14.19   Appliance for preventing tongue thrust. (From Koch G: *Pedodontics: a clinical approach,* Copenhagen, 1991, Munksgaard.)

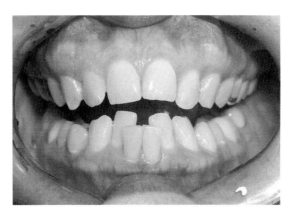

FIG. 14.18   Open bite.

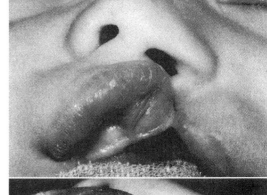

FIG. 14.20   A and B, Cleft lip and palate. (From Proffit WR: *Contemporary orthodontics,* ed 2, St Louis, 1993, Mosby.)

B. Eliminate the habit that is causing the problem, and the teeth will gradually move back into position.

C. Have the dentist construct a special appliance to discourage the offending habit **(FIG. 14.19).**

D. Have the teeth moved orthodontically while the child attempts to eliminate the offending habit (p. 107).

7. Cleft Lip and/or Palate

(FIG. 14.20). Birth defects such as cleft palate and lip are often present. These are caused by genetic transfer from parent to child. Correction of cleft lip and/or palate is highly superior today to that available even a few decades ago. Therapy usually involves a team approach, including a plastic surgeon; oral surgeon; ear, nose, and throat specialist; prosthodontist; speech therapist; psychologist; and others (see Chapter 2). Most large hospitals have a team of these specialists to provide you with answers regarding the overall, long-term care of children with cleft lip and/or palate. Often excellent results can be obtained **(FIG. 14.21).**

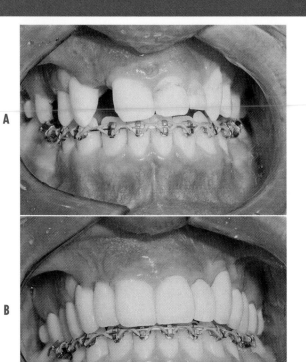

FIG. 14.21 **A and B, Excellent result of treatment for cleft palate.**

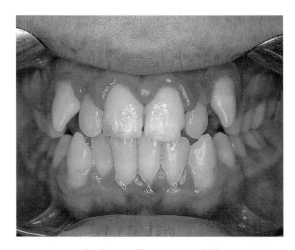

FIG. 14.22 **Bleeding, puffy gums in a child.** (From Regezi JA, Sciubba JJ, Pogrel MA: *Atlas of oral and maxillofacial pathology*, Philadelphia, 2000, WB Saunders.)

8. Gums Red, Puffy, and Bleed Easily

(FIG. 14.22). Numerous conditions cause this problem. Breathing through the mouth most of the time instead of the nose is a common reason for red gums. "Mouth breathing" is usually caused by the child's inability to breathe easily through the nose, and a consultation with an ear, nose, and throat specialist is advisable to determine whether better breathing access can be developed.

Drugs that the child is taking for other conditions may cause red, swollen, irritable gums. Check with your dentist; he or she will be able to determine whether a true gum infection is present.

Some children develop periodontal disease (gum and bone degeneration). The same alternatives exist as those described for an adult with the same condition (p. 134).

9. Child Sucks Thumb or Finger

Most children suck their fingers during early childhood. Some continue beyond the time when the permanent teeth begin to erupt (about age 6). Little damage appears to be caused to developing oral structures by sucking fingers at an early age. However, as the permanent teeth begin to erupt, sucking can cause an open or otherwise incorrect bite, and it should be corrected. Alternatives include the following:

A. Allow the child to continue sucking; sometimes the child stops the habit before any damage is done.
B. Encourage and reward the child for not sucking.
C. Have the dentist construct an oral appliance to discourage the habit.

10. Crooked Teeth

(FIG. 14.23). See Chapter 13 on orthodontics for a complete discussion of this subject. Many preventive or interceptive orthodontic therapies (p. 101) may be accomplished by the dentist during the childhood years to reduce or prevent a need for comprehensive orthodontics at a later time.

11. Child Is Physically or Mentally Handicapped or Is Uncomfortable Permitting Examination and Needs Oral Therapy

Most pediatric dentists and some general dentists provide care for children with these special types of problems. Often, sedation is delivered in the dental office. Healthy chil-

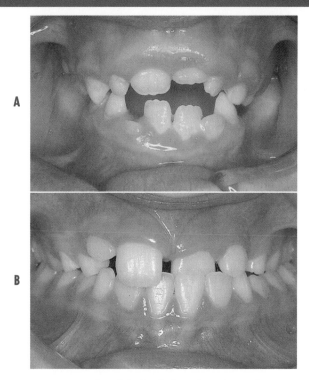

A

B

FIG. 14.23   A and B, Crooked teeth require early correction to prevent the development of more serious problems. (From Millett D, Welbury RR: *Colour guide orthodontics and paediatric dentistry,* 2000, Churchill Livingstone.)

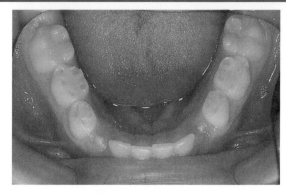

FIG. 14.24   Grinding teeth causes extreme wear. (From Millett D, Welbury RR: *Colour guide orthodontics and paediatric dentistry,* 2000, Churchill Livingstone.)

dren are frequently taken into same-day general anesthetic facilities in hospitals or other locations to allow oral therapy to be completed while the patient is not conscious. When a child is unhealthy, debilitated, or has some type of birth defect, oral therapy may be conducted under general anesthetic in a hospital. This type of therapy usually requires an overnight stay or more. Any time a patient is taken out of the dental office for therapy you can expect that other costs will be incurred.

12. Grinding Teeth

(FIG. 14.24). Bruxism (grinding teeth) (p. 76) is common among children. Sometimes the noise of this habit actually keeps other family members awake at night. Grinding teeth together without food between them wears enamel rapidly and produces flat surfaces on tooth chewing areas.

Because primary (baby) teeth are lost start-

ing at about age 6 and the tooth loss continues for a few years, permanent teeth erupt into place, causing irregularities in the bite relationship, and most children stop grinding their teeth during the mixed dentition (primary and permanent teeth together) stage. However, a few people continue to grind, and they require bruxism therapy at a later time (p. 77). Regardless of age, all persons who grind their teeth excessively should be informed about the destructive nature of the habit and the necessity to discontinue it when they are conscious of their grinding. Adult "bruxers" and "clenchers" need special bite splints (p. 79) to reduce the abnormal wear they are causing their teeth. Such splints usually are not made for children.

13. Teeth Have Peculiar Shape

(FIG. 14.25). Several genetic or disease conditions can cause primary (baby) or permanent teeth to have peculiar shapes (pointed, two fused together, too small or large, etc.). Some of these conditions can be solved by bonding (p. 54) or placing crowns (caps) (p. 146) on the teeth. Conservative, less expensive bonding procedures are almost always advisable over more expensive crowns (caps) during childhood. When full body size has been achieved and oral tissues are more mature, more extensive and expensive therapy such as crowns (caps) may be indicated.

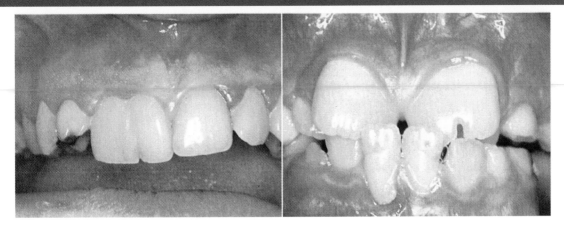

FIG. 14.25 **Peculiarly shaped teeth in children require treatment.** (From Tyldesley WR: *Colour atlas of orofacial diseases,* ed 2, St Louis, 1991, Mosby [Wolfe]. Copyright 1991 by WR Tyldesley.)

A
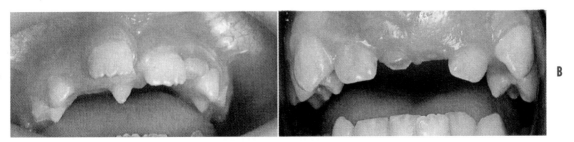
B

FIG. 14.26 **A and B,** **Teeth did not form and therefore did not erupt. Treatment is needed to prevent further problems.** (From Tyldesley WR: *Colour atlas of orofacial diseases,* ed 2, St Louis, 1991, Mosby [Wolfe]. Copyright 1991 by WR Tyldesley.)

Pediatric Dentistry

14. Some Teeth Never Formed or Erupted

(FIG. 14.26). Missing teeth are relatively common, and this condition is usually hereditary. When teeth are missing in a child, it is usually better to place some form of space maintainer (p. 128) that has an acceptable appearance while the child's body matures. At the time of maturation, numerous alternatives are available, including implants (p. 61), fixed prostheses (bridges) (p. 149), or removable prostheses (partial dentures) (p. 162).

15. Primary (Baby) Teeth Discolored

(FIG. 14.27). Several conditions, hereditary or environmental, cause teeth to be discolored. Colors range from brown-orange-yellow to blue-gray. Teeth may be homogeneously discolored, spotted, mottled, or striped, or surface-stained only. Superficial stains can be removed easily and rapidly. However, bodily stain that is internal within the teeth may or may not be removed by bleaching (p. 51). When stains cannot be removed by various bleaching methods, they may be veneered (small pieces of plastic or porcelain bonded to teeth) (p. 55) or crowned (capped) (p. 146). Your dentist can advise you about the specific discolorations on your child's teeth and the treatment alternatives shown in this book.

16. Small, Dark-Colored Grooves or Pits on the Chewing Surfaces

(FIG. 14.28). When the top (chewing) surfaces of molar and premolar (back) teeth form, the tooth substance does not always fuse completely. All molar and premolar teeth have rough-looking chewing surfaces, but some have deep pits and fissures that collect

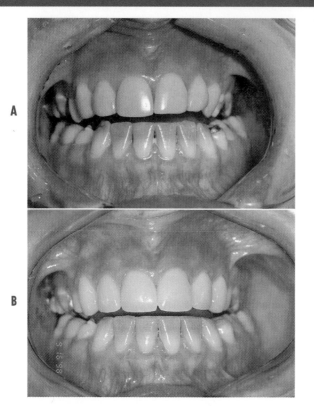

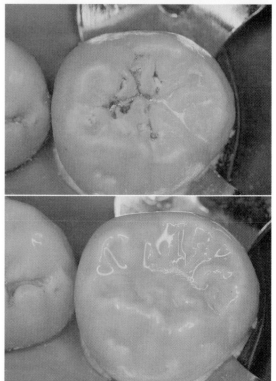

FIG. 14.27   **A,** Discolored teeth in a child caused by drug administration early in life. **B,** Porcelain crowns (caps) have been placed onto the upper anterior teeth for a more natural appearance.

FIG. 14.28   Teeth with dark pits and grooves usually require treatment. **A,** Note stained grooves. **B,** A tooth-colored plastic sealant has been placed.

food debris and cause decay. These suspicious pits and fissures should be sealed with plastic sealants as soon as a dentist or dental hygienist detects them. Sealants prevent decay (dental caries) from forming, by sealing the grooves from bacteria and food debris (p. 182).

WHAT YOUR PEDIATRIC DENTIST OR GENERAL DENTIST CAN DO

Treatment Available

Many of the conditions in children and the treatment provided are similar or the same for adults and are described elsewhere in this book. Each has been referenced in the preceding text of this chapter. Examples are restorations (fillings) (p. 170), bonding (p. 54), crowns (caps) (p. 146), periodontal (gum) therapy (p. 135), and others. Following are some types of treat-

ment that are specific for children and have been mentioned in the previous part of this chapter.

1. Pulpotomy (Removal of a Part of the Dental Pulp [Nerve])

Primary (baby) teeth respond well to removal of a diseased part of the dental pulp (nerve), leaving the healthy portion intact **(FIG. 14.29)**. Permanent teeth do not have this ability. A hole is made in the top of the tooth into the dental pulp, and a portion of the pulp is removed. A sealer is placed on top of the remaining pulp, and a restoration (filling) (p. 170) or a crown (cap) (p. 146) is placed on the tooth.

  A. **Advantages:** The tooth is maintained in service.

  B. **Disadvantages:** Usually a crown (cap) (p. 146) must be placed on the tooth to provide adequate strength. Therefore, the cost is moderate if stainless

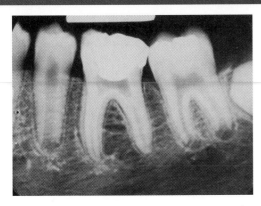

FIG. 14.29 **Pulpotomy removes a part of the dental pulp (nerve) shown in the center tooth.** (From McDonald RE, Avery DR: *Dentistry for the child and adolescent*, ed 7, St Louis, 2000, Mosby.)

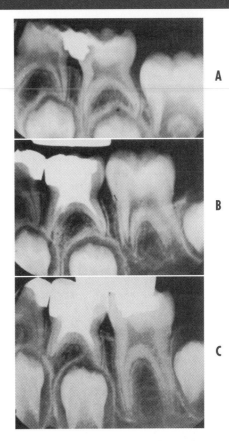

FIG. 14.30 **A to C,** Pulpectomy on a diseased primary (baby) molar. Pulpectomy, root canal filling, and restoration (filling) are shown in the bottom radiograph (x-ray) after healing. (From McDonald RE, Avery DR: *Dentistry for the child and adolescent*, ed 7, St Louis, 2000, Mosby.)

steel is used, and high if ceramic or gold alloy is used.

C. **Risks:** Occasionally a pulpotomy fails, and the tooth must be removed anyway, but the risk is low.

D. **Alternatives:** Alternatives include removal of the tooth and placement of a space maintainer (p. 128), or pulpectomy (removal of all of the pulp) and endodontics (root canal therapy) (p. 40).

E. **Cost:** Although a moderate cost should be expected for the pulpotomy and crown (cap), it may not cost as much as removal of the tooth and placement of a space maintainer.

F. **Result of Nontreatment:** Usually the patient will experience continued and increased pain and infection, and removal of the tooth will be required.

2. Pulpectomy and Endodontic Treatment

(FIG. 14.30). Pulpectomy and endodontic therapy are not common procedures in pediatric dentistry because of their occasional failure versus the success of pulpotomy procedures.

A. **Advantages:** The tooth is maintained in service.

B. **Disadvantages:** The cost for this procedure, followed by the crown (cap) (p. 146), which is necessary for strength, is moderate.

C. **Risks:** Occasionally the procedure fails in children, requiring removal of the tooth.

D. **Alternatives:** Pulpotomy may be accomplished if indicated (p. 124), or the tooth may be extracted, followed by placement of a space maintainer (p. 128).

E. **Cost:** Cost of this procedure plus the crown (cap) (p. 146) required for strength may equal or exceed the cost of tooth removal and placement of a space maintainer.

F. **Result of Nontreatment:** Usually the patient will experience continued and increased pain and infection, and removal of the tooth will be required.

3. Stainless Steel Crown

(FIG. 14.31). Crowns (caps) of several types have been described (p. 146). The stainless

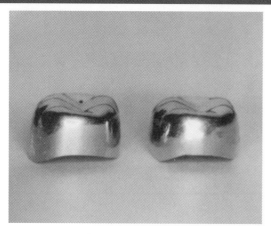

FIG. 14.31   **Stainless steel crowns (caps) are successful and strong, but are not good looking.** (From McDonald RE, Avery DR: *Dentistry for the child and adolescent,* ed 7, St Louis, 2000, Mosby.)

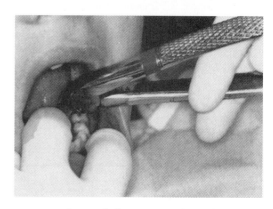

FIG. 14.32   **Removal of primary tooth is unfortunate.** (From Koch G: *Pedodontics: a clinical approach,* Copenhagen, 1991, Munksgaard.)

steel crown (cap) is a type that is commonly used to treat severe tooth destruction in children because its cost is significantly lower than other custom-made crowns (caps). If primary or permanent teeth need crowns (caps), other varieties of crowns (caps) that are more pleasing in appearance (p. 146) or bonding plastic to teeth (p. 54) are more appropriate.

A. **Advantages:** These restorations are relatively strong, inexpensive, reliable, and easily placed by dentists.

B. **Disadvantages:** Stainless steel crowns (caps) have the appearance of polished silver. They are not as long lasting as other custom-made types of crowns (caps) (p. 146); therefore, they are indicated for primary (baby) back teeth, which are not expected to remain in the mouth for a long time. These crowns (caps) contain nickel and chrome, and some persons have sensitivities or allergies to these metals.

C. **Risks:** Occasionally, stainless steel crowns (caps) may come off and be lost or swallowed. New dental caries (decay) can form around the stainless steel crown (cap).

D. **Alternatives:** Some teeth can receive conventional silver alloy or tooth-colored restorations (p. 170) at less expense. Your dentist will advise you if this is possible. However, such restorations are usually much weaker than stainless steel crowns (caps).

E. **Cost:** Because of the time involvement and skill necessary, stainless steel crowns (caps) have a moderate cost.

F. **Result of Nontreatment:** Dental caries (decay) will continue and may eventually destroy the tooth, causing need for its removal. If the placement of the stainless steel crown (cap) was to give a weakened tooth more strength, then lack of its placement may cause fracture and loss of the tooth later.

4. Removal of a Diseased Primary Tooth

(FIG. 14.32). The primary teeth are a specific size and shape. When teeth are prematurely removed, the space occupied by the tooth or teeth is filled by the surrounding teeth, leaving inadequate space for the permanent teeth to erupt. The result is poor occlusion (bite) and unattractive appearance.

A. **Advantages:** The pain is gone soon, and the infection disappears.

B. **Disadvantages:** Often the space occupied by the primary (baby) tooth fills in with other primary teeth, and space is inadequate for the permanent tooth. A space maintainer (p. 128) must be placed if this problem is to be avoided.

C. **Risks:** Minimal surgical risks are involved (p. 92).

D. **Alternatives:** Alternatives include

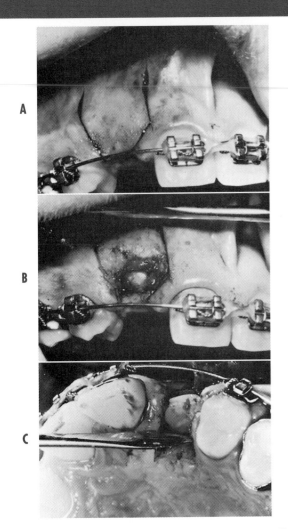

FIG. 14.33   A to C, Surgically assisted eruption: a small incision is made to expose the unerupted tooth and stimulate its eruption. Force may or may not be needed to cause the tooth to erupt. (From Proffit WR, Fields HW Jr: *Contemporary orthodontics*, ed 3, St Louis, 2000, Mosby.)

pulpotomy (p. 124), or pulpectomy (p. 125) and endodontics followed by a crown (cap) (p. 146).

E. **Cost:** Removal of the tooth is low in cost, but the space maintainer needed thereafter is moderate in cost.

F. **Result of Nontreatment:** Nontreatment will result in continuing pain and infection, causing eventual loss of the tooth.

5. Surgically Assisted Eruption

(FIG. 14.33). Making an opening in the gum or bone over a tooth that is slow in erupting can stimulate its entry into the mouth.

A. **Advantages:** The tooth usually erupts faster.

B. **Disadvantages:** There is a minimal cost and slight discomfort.

C. **Risks:** Minimal anesthetic and surgical risk is involved.

D. **Alternatives:** You may wait for the tooth to erupt on its own. Radiographic (x-ray) observation will usually confirm or deny the need for assisted eruption.

E. **Cost:** Minimal cost is involved.

F. **Result of Nontreatment:** Eruption of the underlying permanent tooth will be slower.

6. Assisted Eruption With Orthodontics

(See FIG. 14.11.) If a tooth is shown by radiograph (x-ray) to be in such a location that it cannot erupt naturally, the gum tissue and bone may be opened, allowing access to the tooth. An appliance may be attached to the tooth to guide it into place orthodontically.

A. **Advantages:** The tooth becomes a functioning part of the mouth and provides optimal appearance.

B. **Disadvantages:** Time, effort, some discomfort, and money are required to accomplish this procedure.

C. **Risks:** Occasionally the tooth pulp (nerve) dies during the therapy, requiring root canal therapy (p. 40) and a crown (cap) (p. 146). There are minor normal surgical risks (p. 92).

D. **Alternatives:** You may elect to leave the tooth in place, and it may never erupt, or it may erupt in an improper location. You may also extract the tooth (p. 126).

E. **Cost:** The cost is moderate to high, depending on the complexity of the situation.

F. **Result of Nontreatment:** The appearance of the smile will not be optimal. Some other tooth replacement or orthodontic treatment will probably be needed to fill the space intended for the tooth.

7. Stabilization of Teeth

(See FIG. 14.16.) If a blow or an accident has injured and loosened teeth, some form of splinting or reinforcement of the teeth is often needed while they stabilize.

A. **Advantages:** The teeth cannot move while the bone is healing around them. Faster, more predictable healing is usually observed.

B. **Disadvantages:** Disadvantages include moderate cost and the display of some wires or other splinting material for a period of weeks.

C. **Risks:** The splinting may break away from the teeth, requiring redoing the splint.

D. **Alternatives:** Alternatives include allowing the teeth to stabilize on their own by avoiding any chewing or other activity on the loose teeth.

E. **Cost:** A moderate cost should be expected.

F. **Result of Nontreatment:** Although nonsplinted loose teeth may heal adequately, they can heal in undesirable locations. Splinting provides a predictable outcome.

8. Space Maintainer

(See FIGS. 14.7 and 14.14.) The phrase *space maintainer* is used to describe any form of fixed or removable appliance that fills the space that was created by a missing tooth, thereby saving that space for the expected underlying permanent tooth. Similar devices may be used to reduce tongue thrust (p. 102) or direct jaw growth and movements for a specific need.

A. **Advantages:** The dentition develops with optimal function and appearance.

B. **Disadvantages:** The patient has a fixed or removable appliance in the mouth at all times. If the appliance was placed early in childhood, other such devices may need to be made as body size matures and tooth positions change.

C. **Risks:** Patients may break, lose, or swallow a space maintainer.

D. **Alternatives:** You may elect to let the space remain, with the expected collapse of the bite and resultant lack of space for the permanent tooth.

E. **Cost:** A moderate cost should be expected.

F. **Result of Nontreatment:** It should be expected that adjacent teeth will move to fill the space vacated by the missing tooth, causing poor function and appearance and need for orthodontics (teeth straightening).

SUMMARY

Pediatric dentistry is one of the seven recognized clinical specialties of dentistry. It includes all areas of adult dentistry that may be applied to children. However, it also includes many procedures that are specific to the peculiar needs of primary (baby) teeth and challenges of the developing child. The most significant difference between pediatric and adult dentistry is the need for dentists treating children to understand and practice sound psychological principles to allow children to have positive, relatively pain-free experiences in this important health area. Bad memories of traumatic dental therapy during childhood can influence children negatively and make them reject adequate dental care for life. Find an excellent pediatric or general dentist for your child.

Periodontics
Gums and Bone Surrounding Teeth

Periodontics is an area of dentistry that has been neglected significantly by both dentists and patients. This area of dentistry involves the supporting structures of the teeth, primarily the bone of the jaws and the gum tissue. During adulthood, more teeth are lost to periodontal disease than to dental caries (decay). Why has periodontal therapy been neglected? The most important reason is that disease of the gums and bone progresses slowly and usually is not painful. Most patients do not seek treatment for periodontal disease unless they are motivated by their dentist or dental hygienist. The majority of general dentists emphasize other parts of dental practices, such as restoring teeth (fillings), and they do not motivate patients to seek treatment of periodontal disease.

Although many diseases affect the gums and bone tissues, two are most common: *gingivitis* and *periodontitis*. Gingivitis is simply gum inflammation, not affecting the bone, whereas periodontitis involves degeneration of the bone structure as well as gum inflammation.

Numerous signs and symptoms of periodontal disease (discussed later) are evident to knowledgeable dental patients. Changes in the bone and gums of the jaw may indicate ongoing degeneration and reduction of bone support for teeth and may require professional help. There are dentists who specialize in periodontal therapy (periodontists) in most cities with a significant population; many general dentists also provide periodontal treatment. Patients who think that they have some form of periodontal disease should

ask their general dentist or dental hygienist about the health of their gums and supporting structures. If disease is present beyond the level that the general dentist prefers to treat, the general dentist should refer his or her patient to a periodontist.

WHAT YOU SEE OR FEEL

Conditions, Signs, or Symptoms Related to Periodontics

1. Bleeding From the Gums

(FIG. 15.1). When you eat hard foods, brush your teeth, or use dental floss, blood may come from the gum tissue. If you can localize the area of gum tissue that bleeds, you will see that it is usually redder than the normal pink color of healthy gums. Unless you have done something abusive to your gums, such as eating hard foods, overbrushing, or overflossing, the gums should

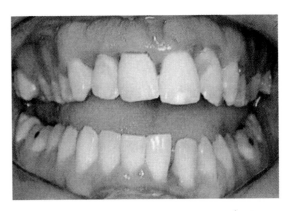

FIG. 15.1   Bleeding gums. (Courtesy Dr. George Bailey, Provo, Utah.)

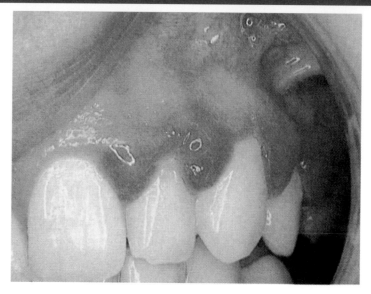

FIG. 15.2   **Red gums may indicate several possible problems.** (From Tyldesley WR: *Colour atlas of orofacial diseases,* ed 2, St Louis, 1991, Mosby [Wolfe]. Copyright 1991 by WR Tyldesley.)

not bleed. Bleeding gums on a regular basis usually indicate that disease is present in the gums and/or bone. The disease is usually gingivitis (gum inflammation) or periodontitis (gum and bone disease). Such bleeding is often upsetting to patients because it does not seem normal or expected. If the bleeding has been present for a short time, the disease process is probably gingivitis. If bleeding has been present for a long time, the disease has probably involved the supporting bone tissue and is periodontitis. Professional care is needed. The following treatment alternatives are available:

A. Dental prophylaxis (p. 134)
B. Scaling teeth (p. 134)
C. Periodontal surgery (p. 135)

2. Red Gums

(FIG. 15.2). Gum tissue that appears to be redder than normal is usually inflamed and engorged with blood, and the gums may bleed when stimulated. Red gums may be caused by numerous conditions, including frequent mouth breathing that leaves a sticky residue on teeth surfaces, leaving food debris on teeth and gum surfaces for prolonged periods, excessive smoking, or drinking of alcoholic beverages, or presence of long-term gum and bone breakdown that have caused increased blood in the gum tissue.

It is difficult for patients to determine the cause of red gums, but a dentist or dental hygienist should be able to tell after an examination. The presence of red gums is usually an indicator of disease activity. One or more of the following methods should be used to treat it:

A. Dental prophylaxis (p. 134)
B. Scaling teeth (p. 134)
C. Periodontal surgery (p. 135)
D. Scaling and polishing teeth followed by application of medications in oral rinses (p. 135)
E. Surgery to correct mouth breathing

3. Creamy, Yellow Substance Comes From Space Between Tooth and Gums; Foul Odor is Present

(FIG. 15.3). Pus discharge from beneath the gums is a nearly sure sign of advanced periodontal disease (gum and bone degeneration) involving the supporting bone tissue. Pus is food debris, dead cells, and microorganisms (bacteria), and is a sign that infection is present. Stimulation of such gums by eating hard foods or cleaning the teeth can cause the infection to be carried to other parts of the body via the blood (bacteremia). Pus discharge can cause disagreeable mouth odors evident to others close enough to smell the breath. When oral disease is present to this degree, it should be treated as soon as possible to avoid further periodontal break-

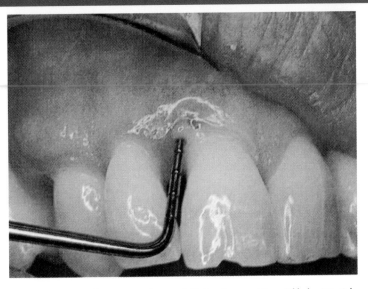

FIG. 15.3   Pus oozing from gum indicates definite disease. (From Tyldesley WR: *Colour atlas of orofacial diseases,* ed 2, St Louis, 1991, Mosby [Wolfe]. Copyright 1991 by WR Tyldesley.)

down. Although such treatment is more difficult than therapy for less advanced periodontal disease, in most cases teeth can still be saved and effectively used for many years. Alternatives for treatment include the following:

A. Scaling teeth (limited treatment potential) (p. 134)

B. Scaling and polishing teeth followed by application of medications in oral rinses (limited treatment potential) (p. 135)

C. Periodontal surgery (p. 135)

D. Tooth extraction (p. 92) and placement of artificial tooth replacements (p. 61)

4. Gums Have Receded From Original Adult Level and Are Unsightly or Sensitive

(FIG. 15.4). Over a lifetime, gum tissue slowly recedes naturally, even with healthy and acceptable periodontal structures. Your gums may have receded naturally, and your mouth may be completely normal and healthy for your age. In such situations the gums are pink and firm, and the teeth are strong and immobile when pressure is applied.

Gum tissue may also recede when periodontal disease is present if it has caused significant bone destruction to reduce tooth support **(FIG. 15.5).** If periodontal disease is present, visible tooth movement may be observed when teeth are moved forward and

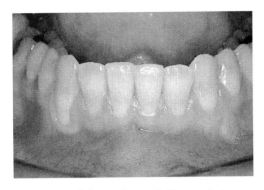

FIG. 15.4   Receded gums (natural). (Courtesy Dr. George Bailey, Provo, Utah.)

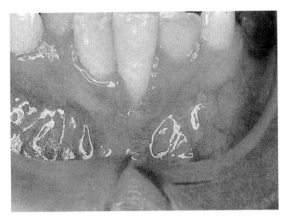

FIG. 15.5   Gum recession as a result of disease. (From Tyldesley WR: *Colour atlas of orofacial diseases,* ed 2, St Louis, 1991, Mosby [Wolfe]. Copyright 1991 by WR Tyldesley.)

Periodontics

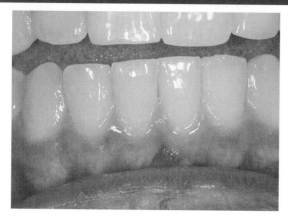

FIG. 15.6   **Normal gum line.**

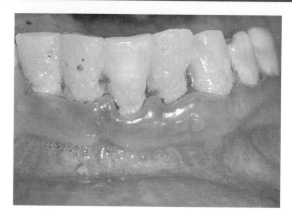

FIG. 15.7   **Food debris collects between teeth.**

backward. Tooth roots will be exposed when gums and bone have receded. Tooth roots are a darker color than tooth crowns (enamel-covered portion of the teeth). The point at which the darker root joins the lighter crown of the tooth is the original location of the gums on the tooth for an adult **(FIG. 15.6)**. Root surfaces may be sensitive to touch, hot and cold foods, or cold air. The two colors of the tooth when the gums have receded may look objectionable to you; therefore, there are two separate potential problems related to receded gums: (A) tooth sensitivity, and (B) disagreeable appearance. The following treatment alternatives are available:

A. Tooth Sensitivity
  (1) Use desensitizing toothpastes for a period of time from weeks to indefinitely (p. 137)
  (2) Place a coat of plastic sealant on the exposed tooth roots to cover and desensitize them (p. 137)
  (3) Place desensitizing chemicals on the exposed tooth roots (p. 137)
  (4) Place desensitizing chemicals on the tooth surfaces and stimulate their penetration onto the exposed tooth roots with iontophoresis (slight electrical current) (p. 137)
  (5) Periodontal surgery, grafting (limited treatment potential) (p. 134)
B. Disagreeable Appearance
  (1) Place crowns (caps) to lengthen tooth appearance and eliminate

the two-color effect on tooth (p. 146)
  (2) Place plastic or porcelain veneers (small pieces of bonded plastic or porcelain that cover the tooth surface) to lengthen tooth appearance and eliminate the two-color effect on tooth (p. 55)
  (3) Place artificial plastic gums (removable)
  (4) Periodontal surgery (limited treatment potential) (p. 135)

5. Food Debris Collects Between Teeth

(FIG. 15.7). Advanced periodontal disease reduces the support of the teeth, and under the stress of biting hard foods, the teeth move. Spaces that develop between the teeth collect food and stagnant mouth debris. This spacing of teeth accompanied by periodontal disease is known as *secondary occlusal trauma* and represents moderate to late periodontal breakdown. Alternatives for treatment include the following:

A. Periodontal surgery followed by crowns (caps) to close the spaces **(FIG. 15.8)**
B. Periodontal surgery followed by orthodontic movement of teeth to close the spaces
C. Scaling and polishing followed by application of medication in oral rinses (limited potential) (p. 135)
D. Splinting the mobile teeth, while filling the spaces with plastic, strengthened with wires or fibers, (p. 127).

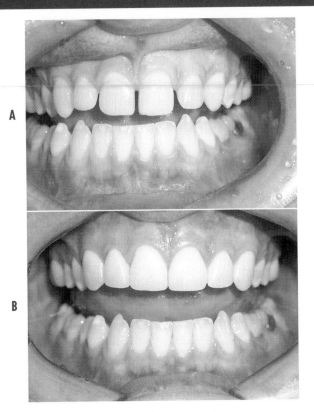

FIG. 15.8 **Closing spaces between teeth with crowns (caps). A,** Before; **B,** after.

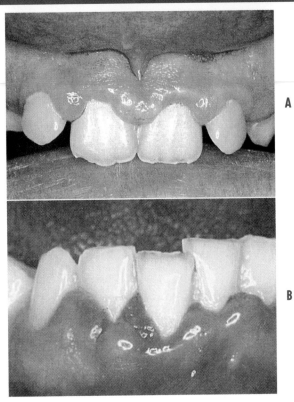

FIG. 15.9 **A and B,** Gums covering the teeth are obviously abnormal and should be corrected. (From Tyldesley WR: *Colour atlas of orofacial diseases,* ed 2, St Louis, 1991, Mosby [Wolfe]. Copyright 1991 by WR Tyldesley.)

6. Mouth Odor (Halitosis)

Unpleasant mouth odor is caused by numerous conditions, including periodontal breakdown, poor or worn out fillings or crowns (caps), digestive system problems, sinus infections, nose disorders, and others. When foul breath is caused by periodontal disease, the factors creating the odor are fermenting food debris, the presence of pus as a result of bone breakdown and pockets formed between the teeth and gums, and long-standing stagnant oral debris that has not been removed. Treatment alternatives include the following:

 A. Improved oral hygiene, including tongue cleaning (p. 179)
 B. Routine scaling and polishing (p. 134)
 C. Periodontal surgery (p. 135)
 D. Scaling and polishing followed by application of medications in oral rinse (p. 135)
 E. New crowns (caps) (p. 146), fillings (p. 170)
 F. Examination and treatment by ear, nose, and throat specialist
 G. Examination and treatment by a general physician

7. Gums Cover Teeth

(FIG. 15.9). A few conditions cause gums to grow excessively and cover the teeth. Gum overgrowth can be caused by administration of various drugs for other health conditions, orthodontic therapy, and other factors. Overgrown gums are usually unsightly and stimulate the patient to seek professional help. Usually the teeth underneath the gum overgrowth are normal and acceptable in appearance. Treatment alternatives include the following:

 A. Periodontal surgery (p. 135)
 B. Improved oral hygiene (p. 176)
 C. Change from the medication causing gum overgrowth

8. Painful Gums

(FIG. 15.10). Pain in or around the gums is usually related to other dental situations, such as

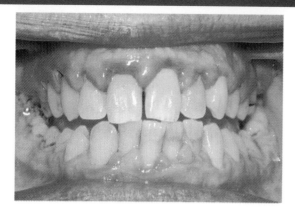

FIG. 15.10 *Patient with painful gums caused by food impaction and long-standing debris.*

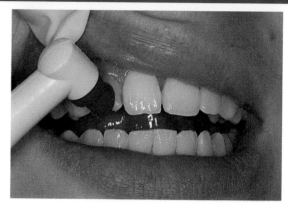

FIG. 15.11 *A rubber cup and abrasive polish used on the teeth usually follow a scaling procedure.*

a dead or dying tooth, food impaction, or other hard foreign objects such as seeds or popcorn shells between the teeth. Pain is not usually present when gingivitis or periodontal disease is in progress. This lack of pain is one of the reasons that diseases of the supporting structures of the teeth (gums and bone) are not treated as soon as desirable.

WHAT YOUR PERIODONTIST, GENERAL DENTIST, OR DENTAL HYGIENIST CAN DO

Treatment Available

1. Dental Prophylaxis

(FIG. 15.11). You have undoubtedly had dental prophylaxis accomplished for you many times. It involves rubbing a sandlike substance on the surfaces of the teeth to clean accumulations of soft debris and/or superficial stains (coffee, tea, cola, chocolate, etc.). A soft rubber cup holding the abrasive material is rotated on the surfaces of the teeth to remove the debris and stain. Most people need this cleaning, along with an oral examination, about once every 6 months, although more or less frequent repetitions may be suggested. Some people build up significant quantities of stains; others do not. A dental hygienist, dentist, or periodontist may perform prophylaxis. Some localities allow dental assistants to clean debris from above the gums.

A. **Advantages:** Surface stains on teeth are removed before they accumulate heavily and are difficult to remove, and during

the examination other developing oral problems can be found before they become severe.

B. **Disadvantages:** Although some people worry about having their teeth cleaned, their concern is unjustified. When accomplished properly, routine dental prophylaxis has no negative results.

C. **Risks:** No risks are involved when the procedure is accomplished correctly on healthy persons.

D. **Alternatives:** None.

E. **Cost:** Very low when compared with the potential cost of neglect.

F. **Result of Nontreatment:** There is significant variation among people. Some have little or no buildup of material on teeth, while others have heavy stain accumulation and tartar buildup (hard deposits on teeth).

2. Scaling Teeth

(FIG. 15.12). Scaling teeth is a routine part of most dental prophylaxis appointments. A scaling instrument (like a hoe or sickle) is placed on the teeth and under the gums to gently remove hard accumulations. Scaling may be accomplished by hand or with mechanical scaling devices. When accomplished properly, scaling produces little or no discomfort.

A. **Advantages:** Routine scaling keeps hard deposits under control and retards the development of periodontal disease. Tartar (hard accumulations on teeth) builds up fast on the teeth of some people and accumulates more

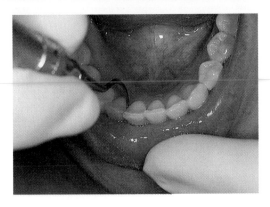

FIG. 15.12 Metal scalers remove hard deposits from teeth relatively easily.

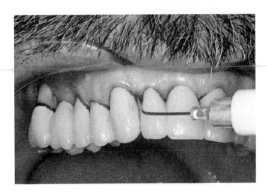

FIG. 15.13 Medications placed under the gums either mechanically or in rinses are very helpful. (Courtesy Dr. George Bailey, Provo, Utah.)

slowly on others. Your dentist or hygienist can tell you the rate of tartar buildup in your own mouth. The timing of your scaling appointments can be set up on your basis of need.

B. **Disadvantages:** None for a normal, healthy individual.

C. **Risks:** None for a normal, healthy individual.

D. **Alternatives:** None.

E. **Cost:** Low if accomplished on a routine basis, but higher if a large accumulation of tartar is allowed to build up.

F. **Result of Nontreatment:** Tartar will build up to the point that occasionally the calcified deposits connect teeth. Periodontal disease and resultant bone loss occurs.

3. Scaling and Prophylaxis Followed by Application of Medications in Oral Rinses

(FIG. 15.13). Many research projects have shown that in some patients with moderate to advanced periodontal disease, scaling and polishing teeth, followed by frequent use of medicated rinses, combined with excellent oral hygiene, can postpone or replace periodontal surgery. This subject is highly controversial, and you will find disagreement among many practitioners. Solutions containing the following chemicals have been used with varying success: chlorhexidine, stannous fluoride, sanguinarine, chlorine dioxide, hydrogen peroxide, and others.

A. **Advantages:** Surgery may be avoided. It may not be necessary to alter the level

of the gums by surgery, and the appearance of the teeth relative to the gums remains the same as it was. If the treatment fails, the more radical treatment—surgery—can always be accomplished.

B. **Disadvantages:** It is difficult to change patient behavior and eliminate poor oral hygiene habits. Patients must direct constant thought and concern toward the cleanliness and treatment of the mouth; several minutes are necessary to accomplish this daily therapy. Thus, treatment (as with other therapy) is not always successful.

C. **Risks:** If periodontal surgery (p. 135) is accomplished, the disease process is usually halted rapidly. If oral medications and rinses are used, time is required to evaluate their effectiveness. During this time the disease process could be continuing, and the postponement could make the periodontal disease worse.

D. **Alternatives:** Periodontal surgery (p. 135) is the only major alternative.

E. **Cost:** The cost of this therapy is relatively low, but it continues for an indefinite period.

F. **Result of Nontreatment:** The periodontal disease continues to worsen, and the teeth are eventually lost.

4. Periodontal Surgery (Gums Only)

(FIG. 15.14). Some periodontal techniques involving gums only are gingivectomy (removal of

Periodontics

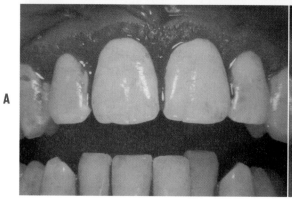
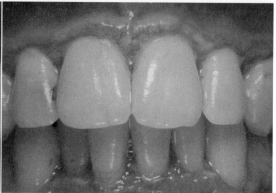

FIG. 15.14 **A,** The gingivectomy being performed on this person may look worse than it is. **B,** This surgery heals rapidly.

selected gum tissue), gingivoplasty (recontouring gums), gingival curettage (removal of inside lining of gums), soft-tissue grafting (moving gum tissue from one site to another), mucogingival surgery (changing position of various parts of gums), apically repositioned flaps (moving portions of gums), and others. In some situations the bone supporting the teeth is in excellent health, and the soft tissue (gums) has some form of defect or disease. This type of periodontal surgery causes less discomfort and heals faster than the surgery involving bone tissue. Soft-tissue periodontal surgery can be used to reduce the amount of gum tissue showing, thus uncovering teeth. It can also be used to move small pieces of tissue from other parts of the mouth or another donor site to fill in areas where the gums are not adequate (grafting). With curettage, a form of soft-tissue surgery, a sharp scaler or a laser is introduced in the space between the tooth and the gum to remove or shrink the soft tissue and reduce the depth of the pocket between the gum and the tooth.

A. **Advantages of Periodontal Surgery (Gums Only):** The procedure is relatively simple, without significant discomfort, and the surgical site heals rapidly (days to weeks). Gum-tissue deficiencies or excess gum tissue can thereby be corrected.

B. **Disadvantages:** Most people experience slight discomfort, and care must be taken to allow adequate healing.

C. **Risks:** Well-accomplished periodontal

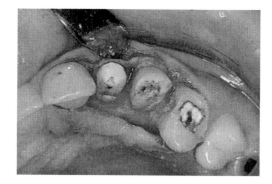

FIG. 15.15 **Osseous (bone) surgery recontours the supportive bone and allows the gums to heal. If you need it, get it, or you will lose your teeth.** (Courtesy Dr. George Bailey, Provo, Utah.)

soft-tissue surgery has few risks, mostly for persons with bleeding problems or anesthetic allergies.

D. **Alternatives:** When bone degeneration is not present, periodontal surgery on the gums is the only acceptable alternative.

E. **Cost:** Moderate cost should be expected.

F. **Result of Nontreatment:** The condition will continue as it is or become progressively worse.

5. Periodontal Surgery (Gums and Bone)

(FIG. 15.15). After periodontal disease has progressed for months to years, the underlying bone tissue will have degenerated. Craters and defects are present in the bone (FIG. 15.16) and will require surgical correction. Numerous methods are used, including the following:

i. The soft tissue (gums) is reflected away

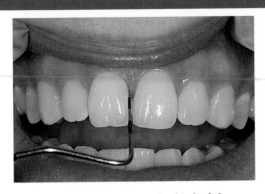

FIG. 15.16 Probes demonstrate the depth of the gum sulcus. It should only be ¹⁄₁₆ to ⅛ inch deep.

from the bone temporarily, and the bone is reshaped or recontoured. The gums are replaced and healing takes place.

ii. The gums are reflected away from the bone temporarily, and the bone defects are filled with bone-grafting material, which can be:

- Bone from other locations in the patient
- Bone from other persons, or
- Artificial bone

iii. The gums are removed temporarily from the bone, and the bone defects are located and filled in one of the ways described immediately above (ii). Sometimes a fabric membrane is placed over the graft site to improve the potential for solid bone to fill the defects (guided tissue regeneration). The gums are replaced, and healing takes place. This surgery may require removal of the fabric membrane at a later time.

All of these procedures are relatively complex and require time for the surgery, which is usually accomplished in the periodontist's or general dentist's office, followed by a healing period. Some discomfort is to be expected. This type of therapy is the only acceptable one for some types of periodontal disease.

A. **Advantages:** The bone defects and soft-tissue defects may be corrected rapidly at the same time.

B. **Disadvantages:** The procedures require time and effort, and some discomfort must be expected. Occasionally the surgery is not successful, and other surgical procedures are required. Teeth can be sensitive for a time after

surgery. The appearance of the gums will be different. Less gum tissue will show, and sometimes teeth can appear objectionably long. Consult with your dentist about your specific situation and the potential results.

C. **Risks:** Healthy persons have no risks. Those with bleeding problems or anesthetic allergies have a slight risk and practitioners should control these well.

D. **Alternatives:** Some practitioners advocate scaling and prophylaxis followed by application of medications in oral rinses. However, in the middle to late stages of periodontal disease, the success potential is very limited. Teeth may be extracted and artificial teeth and gums placed in the mouth; in the late stages of periodontal disease, this more radical option may be the best one for some people when potential for surgical success is limited.

E. **Cost:** These procedures are difficult and time-consuming, and thus are moderately expensive.

F. **Result of Nontreatment:** The periodontal disease process will continue, and teeth will eventually be extracted.

6. Desensitization of Teeth

(FIG. 15.17). Many conditions cause sensitivity of teeth, including diet, digestive system problems, some foods, regurgitation (vomiting), receding gums, and shrinkage of gum tissue caused by periodontal surgery. This condition is irritating to patients but causes little or no harm to teeth or gums. Among the methods used to desensitize teeth are the following:

- Use of desensitizing toothpastes
- Sealing the surface of the tooth with various adhesives to prevent future entrance of the sensitizing agent into the tooth
- Placement of chemicals such as fluoride on the teeth to reduce or eliminate the sensitivity
- Use of fluoride in trays
- Iontophoresis (electrical stimulation of chemicals into the teeth surface)

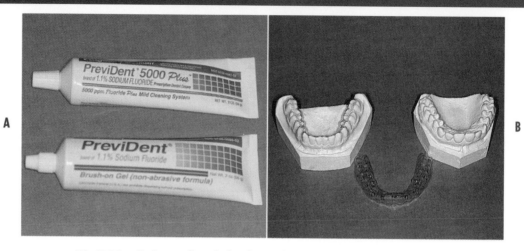

FIG. 15.17 **A,** Strong fluoride brush-on gels. **B,** Fluoride gel applied in trays desensitize teeth.

A. **Advantages:** Reduction or elimination of tooth pain.
B. **Disadvantages:** You must take the time and pay someone to desensitize the teeth.
C. **Risks:** None except for persons with allergies or other health problems.
D. **Alternatives:** None, except to crown (cap) the teeth or remove them, which would be foolish except in extreme cases.
E. **Cost:** The cost is relatively low and is spread over time.
F. **Result of Nontreatment:** The teeth remain sensitive except in cases in which the cause of sensitivity, such as a certain food or drink, is eliminated.

SUMMARY

Just as a sound foundation is important to a house, the teeth must have a sound foundation of bone and gum tissue. If this foundation is not present, the teeth will be lost eventually. Good oral hygiene (p. 176) is not difficult to accomplish, and combined with routine oral examinations (every 6 months or more frequently), dental prophylaxis, and scaling as needed, most people do not develop periodontal disease. Treatment of periodontal disease is often neglected; therefore, encourage your dentist and dental hygienist to tell you if they see any signs of periodontal breakdown.

CHAPTER 16

Prosthodontics, Fixed
Crowns (Caps) or Bridges Cemented Onto Teeth

Most of the tooth structure that is observable when looking into the mouth is dental enamel. It is a coating about ⅟₁₆ inch (1 to 1.5 mm) thick that covers the internal portion of the tooth, the dentin (FIG. 16.1). Enamel is the hardest substance in the body, and it protects the tooth from injury. Enamel is not present on the tooth root (the portion of the tooth that is in the bone). The portion of the tooth that protrudes into the mouth is called the clinical crown.

When a large portion of the enamel covering the clinical crown has been destroyed by dental caries (decay), has had fillings, is broken or worn, or is defective in other ways, the enamel layer must be replaced with an artificial crown (cap). Artificial crowns

(caps) fit onto prepared (trimmed) teeth like a stocking cap fits on your head. Crowns (caps) are cemented into place, replacing the enamel and some of the dentin (FIG. 16.2).

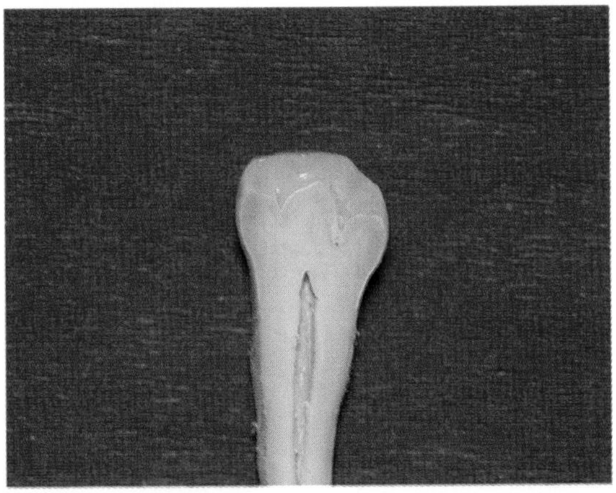

If a single tooth or a few teeth are missing, the enamel may be removed from teeth adjacent to the space, and a fixed prosthesis (fixed bridge) may be cemented into place to fill the space created by the tooth removal (FIG. 16.3).

Crowns (caps) and fixed prostheses range from simple to highly complex, depending on the situation. They may be metal alone, metal with tooth-colored porcelain fired over it, or, in some situations, porcelain, ceramic, or plastic alone. Most dentists delegate the construction of crowns (caps) and fixed prostheses to dental laboratory technicians, while the preparation (trimming) of the teeth and seating of the crowns (caps) or prostheses are accomplished by the dentist and the clinical staff.

Costs for crowns (caps) and fixed prostheses are higher than most other oral treatment because of the clinical skills necessary, the expense for significant laboratory time, the cost of metals, and long-term follow-up.

Most general dentists accomplish simple to moderately complex fixed prostheses. However, complex clinical situations are often referred to prosthodontists, who have had more education and/or experience in this area.

This chapter discusses clinical conditions that you will recognize and lists types of treatment that your general dentist or prosthodontist can provide.

FIG. 16.1 **This tooth has been cut in half. Note the thin layer of enamel on the outside of the top of the tooth. This enamel is removed when a crown (cap) is made for the tooth.**

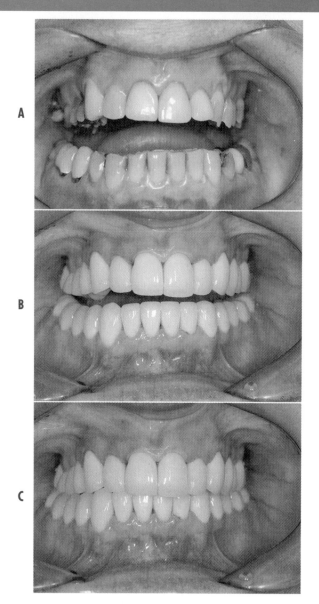

FIG. 16.2   **A,** Worn, decayed, and discolored teeth.
B, Teeth restored with crowns (caps), bite open. **C,** Bite
closed into chewing position.

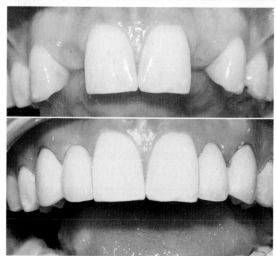

FIG. 16.3   **A,** Two missing upper lateral incisors. **B,** Fixed
prostheses (bridges), attached to the canines (eye teeth)
and replacing the lateral incisors, are undetectable.

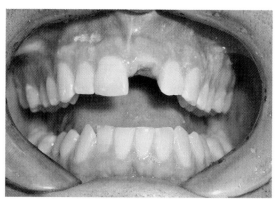

FIG. 16.4   A missing front tooth is unacceptable in
appearance to most people.

WHAT YOU SEE OR FEEL

Conditions, Signs, or Symptoms Related to Fixed Prosthodontics

1. One Missing Tooth

(FIG. 16.4). If one tooth is missing in the front
of the mouth, the situation is unsightly, and
most persons prefer to have the space filled
with an artificial tooth as soon as possible. A
missing tooth in the back portion of the
mouth, in a location where it is not observable, may or may not require replacement because of appearance. However, most teeth
that are removed, regardless of where they
were located in the mouth, can cause
significant movement of surrounding teeth
and collapse of the occlusion (bite) **(FIG. 16.5).**
If your missing tooth has caused an unsightly
space in your smile, you may want to replace
it soon; but if one of your back teeth was removed, you should discuss the potential collapse of the bite with your dentist before
choosing from your alternatives. Usually, you
have the following treatment alternatives:

A. Fixed prosthesis (traditional bridge involving at least one tooth on each side
   of space as abutment teeth) (p. 149)

B. Fixed prosthesis (Maryland bridge) (less
   prepared [less trimmed] teeth on each

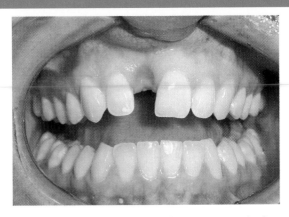

FIG. 16.5   Don't wait too long! This person waited a few years before attempting to replace the tooth, and the result (collapse) is evident.

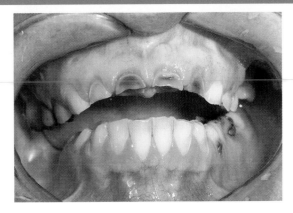

FIG. 16.6   This person has a poor appearance and diminished self-esteem.

side of the space, with conservative bridge holding a false tooth and usually leaving the front portion of the abutment [supporting] teeth intact) (p. 152)

C. Cantilever fixed prosthesis (traditional bridge involving one or more teeth on one side of space, only as abutments) (p. 151)

D. Removable partial denture (all plastic) (p. 162)

E. Removable partial denture (traditional metal and plastic) (p. 162)

F. Removable partial denture, precision or semi-precision (plastic and metal fitted to crowns [caps]) (p. 162)

G. Implant(s) with crown(s) (caps) or prosthesis fixed on top to replace teeth (p. 72)

H. Implant(s) with removable partial denture placed on top of them (p. 70)

2. A Few Missing Teeth

(FIG. 16.6). A few missing teeth usually cause an unsightly appearance and some loss of function. Almost always, the removal of a few teeth causes a collapse of the occlusion (bite) over a period of months to years **(FIG. 16.7)**. Often the loss of a few teeth has been caused by trauma or ongoing periodontal (gum) disease, in which case periodontal therapy must be accomplished before fixed prostheses are placed. When a few teeth have been missing for months to years, significant soft-tissue and

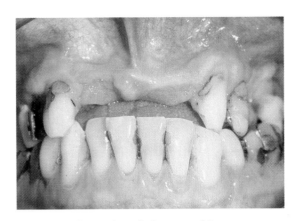

FIG. 16.7   Observe how the lower teeth have over-erupted into the space on the upper jaw.

bone shrinkage usually have occurred. All of the conditions described influence the desirability or acceptability of the following treatment alternatives:

A. Fixed prosthesis (traditional bridge involving at least one tooth on each side of space as abutment teeth) (p. 149)

B. Fixed prosthesis (Maryland bridge) (less prepared [less trimmed] teeth on each side of the space, with conservative bridge holding a false tooth and usually leaving the front portion of the abutment teeth intact) (p. 152)

C. Cantilever fixed prosthesis (traditional bridge involving one or more teeth on one side of space only as abutments) (p. 151)

D. Removable partial denture (all plastic) (p. 162)

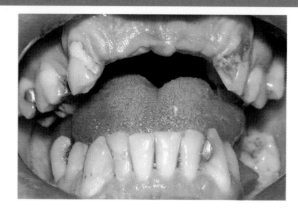

FIG. 16.8 **Many missing teeth can be restored well with fixed prostheses.**

E. Removable partial denture (traditional metal and plastic) (p. 162)
F. Removable partial denture, precision or semi-precision (plastic and metal is fitted to crowns [caps]) (p. 162)
G. Implant(s) with crown(s) (caps) or prosthesis fixed on top to replace teeth (p. 72)
H. Implant(s) with removable partial denture placed on top of them (p. 70)

3. Many Missing Teeth

(FIG. 16.8). Almost always, many missing teeth cause an unsightly appearance, moderate loss of function, and eventual collapse of the occlusion (bite). Periodontal disease may have caused the loss of teeth and may need treatment before a fixed prosthesis is placed. Significant soft-tissue and bone shrinkage can be present also. All of the above conditions influence the acceptability of the following treatment alternatives:

A. Fixed prosthesis (traditional bridge involving at least one tooth on each side of space as abutment teeth) (p. 149)
B. Fixed prosthesis (Maryland bridge) (less prepared [less trimmed] teeth on each side of the space, with conservative bridge holding a false tooth and usually leaving the front portion of the abutment teeth intact) (p. 152)
C. Cantilever fixed prosthesis (traditional bridge involving one or more teeth on one side of space only as abutments) (p. 151)

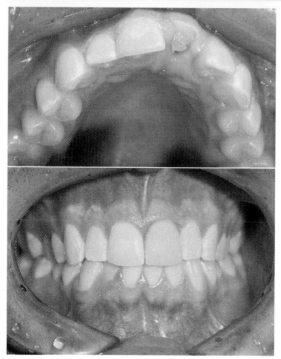

FIG. 16.9 **A,** This tooth is severely broken. **B,** A crown (cap) was placed on the remaining reconstructed tooth root.

D. Removable partial denture (all plastic) (p. 162)
E. Removable partial denture (traditional metal and plastic) (p. 162)
F. Removable partial denture, precision or semi-precision (plastic and metal fitted to crowns [caps]) (p. 162)
G. Implant(s) with crown(s) (caps) or prosthesis fixed on top to replace teeth (p. 72)
H. Implant(s) with removable partial denture placed on top of them (p. 70)

4. Broken or Cracked Tooth (Teeth)

(FIG. 16.9). When a significant amount of tooth structure has broken off, a crown (cap) is usually the strongest and most esthetic in appearance for restoration of the tooth. However, several treatment alternatives are also possible:

A. Crown (cap) (p. 146)
B. Tooth-colored restoration (filling) (p. 173)
C. Metallic restoration (filling) (p. 170)
D. Extraction (p. 92)
E. Fixed (p. 149) or removable prostheses (bridges) (p. 162)

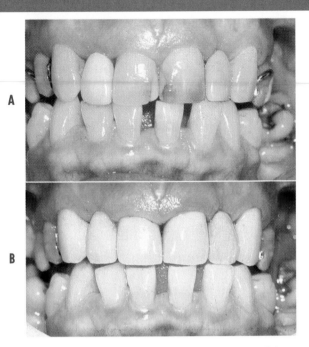

FIG. 16.10 **A,** Dental decay has produced an unsightly appearance in the upper front teeth. **B,** The condition was corrected with six crowns (caps).

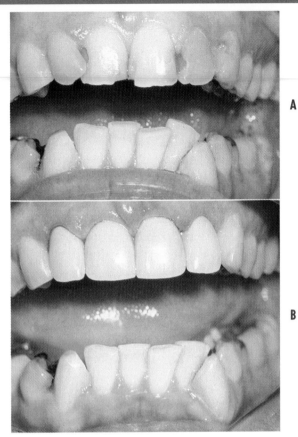

FIG. 16.11 **A,** When old fillings degenerate seriously, the best alternative often is crowns (caps). **B,** Four crowns (caps) were placed on the upper front teeth.

5. Teeth With Large Dental Caries (Decayed Areas)

(FIG. 16.10). Significant destruction of tooth structure by dental caries is usually repaired best by placing a crown (cap), but more conservative measures may be possible also:

- A. Crown (cap) (p. 146)
- B. Tooth-colored restoration (filling) (p. 173)
- C. Metallic restoration (filling) (p. 170)
- D. Extraction (p. 92)
- E. Fixed (p. 49) or removable prostheses (bridges) (p. 162)

6. Teeth With Large Defective Fillings

(FIG. 16.11). Placement of large fillings in teeth usually requires removal of a significant portion of tooth structure, and replacement with new fillings is often not possible. Crowns (caps) are usually the strongest and most esthetically acceptable of the following alternatives:

- A. Crown (cap) (p. 146)
- B. Tooth-colored restoration (filling) (p. 173)
- C. Metallic restoration (filling) (p. 170)

- D. Extraction (p. 92)
- E. Fixed (p. 149) or removable prostheses (bridges) (p. 162)

7. Crooked Teeth

(FIG. 16.12). Many times, slightly to moderately crooked teeth can be straightened and improved in appearance by placing restorations (fillings, bonding, veneers) or crowns (caps). The following treatment alternatives are possible:

- A. Crown (cap) (p. 146)
- B. Tooth-colored restoration (filling) (p. 173)
- C. Bonding (p. 54)
- D. Veneers (p. 55)
- E. Orthodontics (straightening) (p. 107)
- F. Extraction (p. 92)
- G. Fixed (p. 149) or removable prostheses (bridges) (p. 162)

Prosthodontics, Fixed

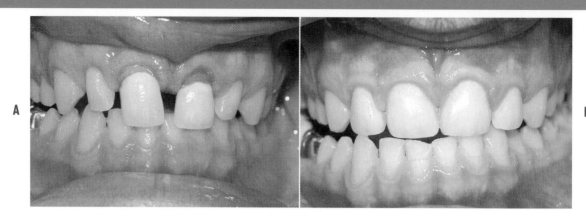

FIG. 16.12 **A,** Crooked teeth. **B,** Unsightly appearance and poor function solved with four new crowns (caps) on upper front teeth.

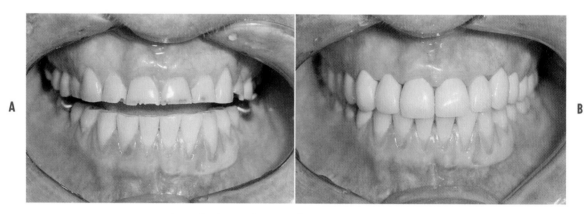

FIG. 16.13 **A,** Worn, broken teeth. **B,** Replacement with pleasing new crowns (caps).

8. Previously Placed Crown(s) (Caps) or Fixed Prostheses (Bridges) Have Foul Taste or Emit Odor

(FIG. 16.13). Dental decay (caries) or periodontal (gum and bone) disease may occur around crowns (caps) or fixed prostheses (fixed bridges), causing a foul taste and/or odor from the crowns (caps) or prostheses (bridges). Additionally, a fixed prosthesis (bridge) may become loose on one end and still remain in the mouth, trapping food debris that can cause dental caries (decay) under the loose end. Usually, a foul taste and/or odor will result from this condition, and its elimination usually requires some of the following therapy:

    A. Periodontal (gum and bone) therapy (p. 135)

    B. New crowns (caps) and fixed prostheses (bridges) (p. 146)

    C. Repair of crowns (caps) or fixed pros-

theses (bridges) currently in place (p. 153)

9. Crowns (Caps) or Fixed Prostheses (Bridges) Are Large, Bulky, Wrong Color, or Otherwise Unpleasing in Appearance

(FIG. 16.14). Your oral conditions may have changed since the initial placement of crowns (caps) or a fixed prosthesis, thereby causing an unpleasing appearance, or they may have been unacceptable to you at the time of initial placement. Probably the only acceptable alternative is to redo the crowns (caps) or fixed prostheses. There is a minor chance that repair can be done without redoing the restorations, as follows:

    A. New crowns (caps) or fixed prostheses (bridges) (p. 146)

    B. Repair of the crowns (caps) or fixed prostheses (bridges) currently in place (p. 153)

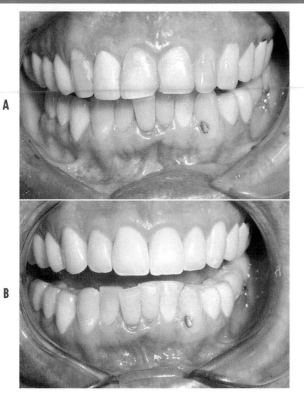

FIG. 16.14   **A,** Worn, chipped restoration. **B,** What a difference six new crowns (caps) make on these upper front teeth.

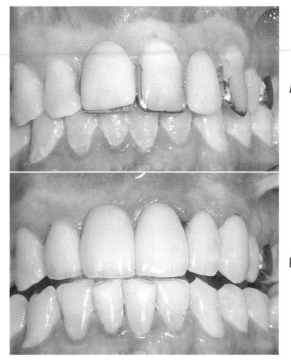

FIG. 16.15   **A,** These old crowns (caps) on the upper front teeth are broken and too bulky. **B,** New crowns (caps) create a much better appearance.

10. Broken Crowns (Caps) or Fixed Prostheses (Bridges)

(FIG. 16.15). The tooth-colored portion of crowns (caps) or fixed prostheses can break away from underlying metal, or in some cases the metal understructure can fracture. Occasionally, repair can be accomplished, but most often replacement of the restorations is necessary. The following are therapy alternatives:

A. New crowns (caps) or fixed prostheses (bridges) (p. 146)

B. Repair of crowns (caps) or fixed prostheses (bridges) currently in place (p. 153)

11. Pain When Biting Force Is Applied on Crowns (Caps) or Fixed Prostheses

(FIG. 16.16). Previously treated teeth may cause pain if the pulp (nerve) is dead or dying (p. 37). Fixed prostheses (fixed bridges) that are loose on one end may cause pain on chewing. Dental caries (decay) may be present. The following alternatives are available:

A. Endodontic therapy through a small

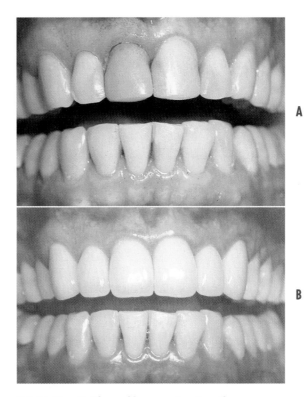

FIG. 16.16   **A,** These old crowns (caps) on the upper front teeth are painful because of leakage and dental caries (decay). **B,** The six new crowns (caps) corrected the problem.

hole in crown (cap) or fixed prostheses (p. 40)

B. Repair of crowns (caps) or fixed prostheses (bridges) currently in place (p. 153)

C. New crowns (caps) (p. 146) or fixed prostheses (bridges) (p. 149)

WHAT YOUR PROSTHODONTIST OR GENERAL DENTIST CAN DO

Treatment Available

1. Single Crown (Cap), Metal

(FIG. 16.17). In the past, this was the only type of crown (cap) available. The involved tooth is trimmed down, removing most of the outside layer (enamel). This prepared (trimmed) tooth looks similar to a miniature normal tooth. An impression (mold) of the prepared tooth is made, and a model is constructed in a plasterlike material by a dental laboratory technician. On that model is made a wax form of the tooth, replacing the missing tooth structure. The wax form or pattern is placed inside a plasterlike substance (investment), and the wax is "burned out" with heat, leaving a void inside the investment. A metal alloy is melted and cast into the void in the investment, thus reproducing in metal the exact shape of the original wax pattern. This technique is known as lost wax casting. Although all dentists learn the technique in dental school, most of them delegate crown (cap) construction to dental laboratory technicians. The fee for the laboratory portion of the crown (cap) is included in the dentist's fee. While the crown (cap) is being made, the patient wears a temporary crown (cap) that is made of plastic. The crown (cap) is cemented onto the trimmed tooth using various dental cements.

A. **Advantages:** This dental restoration is among the longest lasting and strongest services in dentistry. Many types of gold alloy crowns (caps) wear during chewing at about the same rate as natural tooth enamel, which causes less wear on opposing teeth.

B. **Disadvantages:** The only significant disadvantage of metal crowns (caps) is

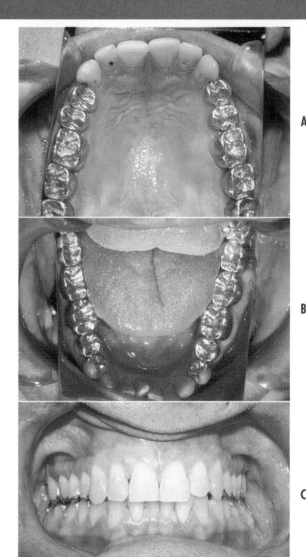

FIG. 16.17 Gold crowns (caps) are the longest-lasting restoration in dentistry. **A** and **B,** Gold alloy crowns (caps) and onlays viewed from the chewing surface. **C,** Relatively good appearance from the front of the mouth.

the display of metal in the mouth. This is unacceptable to some people and limits the use of metal crowns (caps) to the back part of the mouth, where they are not readily visible.

C. **Risks:** There are very few risks with metal crowns (caps). Occasionally, prepared (trimmed) teeth are injured inadvertently during the trimming procedure, and the tooth may require root canal therapy (p. 40) during the crown (cap) treatment or after the crown (cap) has been cemented into the mouth. Infrequently, persons may have allergies to the metal elements used in the crown (cap), and a discussion of this possibility should be a part of the decision process before you accept the dentist's treatment plan for crowns (caps). If necessary, crowns (caps) without metal can be made for some situations (p. 147).

D. **Alternatives:** If a crown (cap) is needed and metal is not indicated, the following procedures are available:
   1. Porcelain crown (cap) with nonvisible metal underneath (porcelain fused to metal) (p. 147)
   2. Plastic (resin) crown (cap) with non-visible metal underneath (p. 149)
   3. Ceramic crown (cap) without any metal (p. 147)
   4. Plastic (resin) crown (cap) without any metal (p. 149)
   5. A patch or repair of the tooth for an interim time with traditional filling materials (p. 170)

E. **Cost:** Metal crowns (caps) are expensive compared with typical restorations (fill-ings), and a crown (cap) will cost three to eight times more than a typical metal or tooth-colored restoration (filling). Usually the various types of crowns (caps) do not vary significantly in cost.

F. **Result of Nontreatment:** Assuming that the need for crowns (caps) has been diagnosed correctly, teeth will continue to degenerate, crack, break off, and decay until tooth removal becomes necessary.

2. Single Crown (Cap), Porcelain-Fused-to-Metal (PFM)

(FIG. 16.18). PFM crowns (caps) are thin metal crowns (caps) that have tooth-colored porcelain fused (baked) by heat onto the metal. These are the most commonly used crowns (caps) in dentistry today.

A. **Advantages:** When constructed properly, PFM crowns (caps) are among the most beautiful tooth restorations in dentistry, and some are nearly indiscernible from natural teeth.

B. **Disadvantages:** The porcelain placed on PFM crowns (caps) is abrasive to opposing natural tooth structure and metal crowns (caps), and wear of opposing natural teeth and metal crowns (caps) can be expected. Infrequently, porcelain can be fractured from the underlying metal during chewing or in an accident that delivers force to the crown (cap).

C. **Risks:** The only significant risks are wear of opposing teeth over years of service, and the slight chance that root canal therapy (p. 40) could be needed at a later time.

D. **Alternatives:** See Single Crown (Cap), Metal (p. 146).

E. **Cost:** See Single Crown (Cap), Metal (p. 146).

F. **Result of Nontreatment:** See Single Crown (Cap), Metal (p. 146).

3. Single Crown (Cap), Ceramic (No Metal)

(FIG. 16.19). There are at least two reasons why patients might need or prefer crowns (caps) that do not contain any metal: (1) They have known or suspected sensitivities or allergies to the metal elements in all metal or porcelain-fused-to-metal (PFM) crowns (caps), and (2) they prefer the slightly more lifelike appearance of all-ceramic crowns (caps) over PFM crowns (caps).

A. **Advantages:** The appearance of ceramic crowns (caps) may be slightly better than that of porcelain crowns (caps) containing metal, and, as the gums shrink over a period of years, metal or discoloration will not be observed at the gum line. Ceramic crowns (caps) without metal do not have significant sensitivity or allergy potential compared with metal crowns (caps).

B. **Disadvantages:** They are significantly weaker than PFM crowns (caps).

C. **Risks:** See Single Crown (Cap), Metal (p. 146) for overall risks of crowns (caps). The only additional risk is the reduced strength of ceramic crowns (caps).

D. **Alternatives:** See Single Crown (Cap), Metal (p. 146).

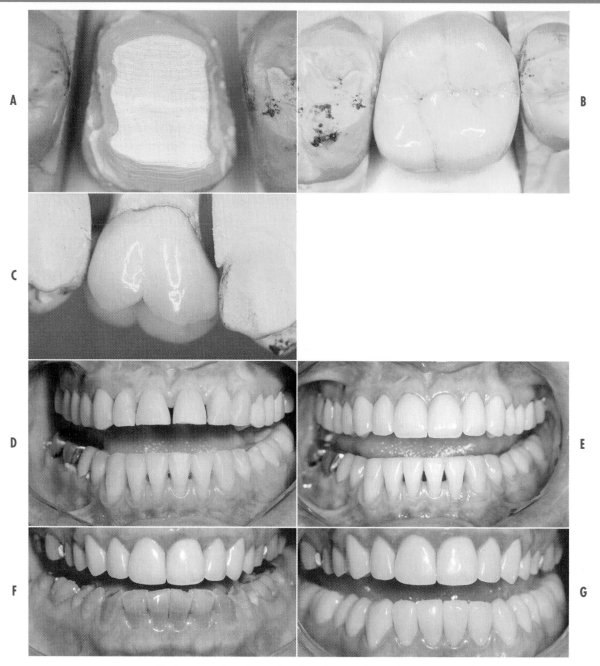

FIG. 16.18 Single crowns (caps), porcelain fused to metal, are the most commonly used crowns (caps) in dentistry. **A,** Model of a tooth prepared for a crown (cap). **B** and **C,** The crown (cap) on a laboratory model. **D** and **E,** Before and after single crowns (caps) were placed on upper front teeth. **F** and **G,** Before and after crowns (caps) were placed on the lower front teeth.

E. **Cost:** See Single Crown (Cap), Metal (p. 146).

F. **Result of Nontreatment:** See Single Crown (Cap), Metal (p. 146).

4. Single Crown (Cap), Plastic (Resin) on Metal

(FIG. 16.20). Crowns (caps) of resin on metal are not popular, but occasionally dentists will suggest them. The only significant differences between resin on metal and porcelain-fused-to-metal are that resin is weaker, and resin does not wear opposing teeth.

5. Single Crown (Cap), Plastic (Resin) (No Metal)

Resin crowns (caps) are similar in appearance to those in Fig. 16.20. They are not popular. They are similar to ceramic crowns (caps)

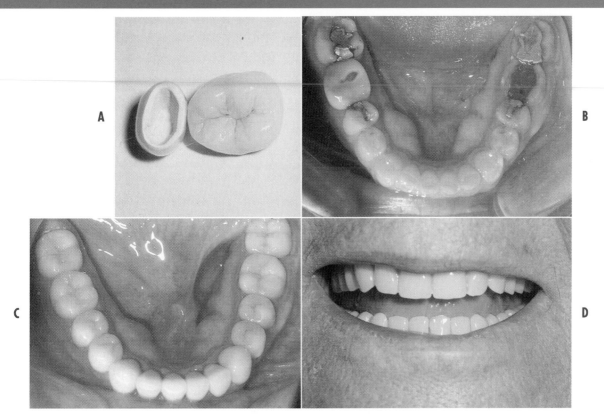

FIG. 16.19 **Some people need all-ceramic crowns (caps) because of metal sensitivities. Others prefer the beautiful appearance of all-ceramic crowns (caps). However, they are somewhat weaker than porcelain-fused-to-metal crowns (caps). A,** Two all-ceramic **crowns (caps). B, C,** and **D,** Before, with metal; after, with all-ceramic crowns (caps).

(p. 147), but they do not wear opposing teeth.

6. Fixed Prosthesis (Fixed Bridge), Traditional (Three or More Tooth Units Involved)

(FIG. 16.21). Other than single crowns (caps), this is the portion of fixed prosthodontics that most people know about. When a patient has one or more missing teeth, they can be replaced often by preparing (trimming down) one or more of the teeth adjacent to the space on each side and spanning the gap with lifelike artificial teeth connected to the prepared (trimmed down) natural teeth. The resultant bridge is cemented into place, and it looks and feels similar to natural teeth.

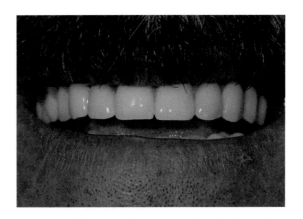

FIG. 16.20 **This patient has no natural teeth; the teeth you see are plastic bonded to metal, supported by dental implants.**

A. **Advantages:** These tooth replacements appear and function similar to natural teeth. They remain in the mouth at all times. However, they are cleaned with special care and somewhat different methods than natural teeth.

B. **Disadvantages:** The trimmed down natural teeth to which the bridge is attached (abutments) must carry the load for their own position in the mouth in addition to the load of the missing teeth. Sometimes they can be over-

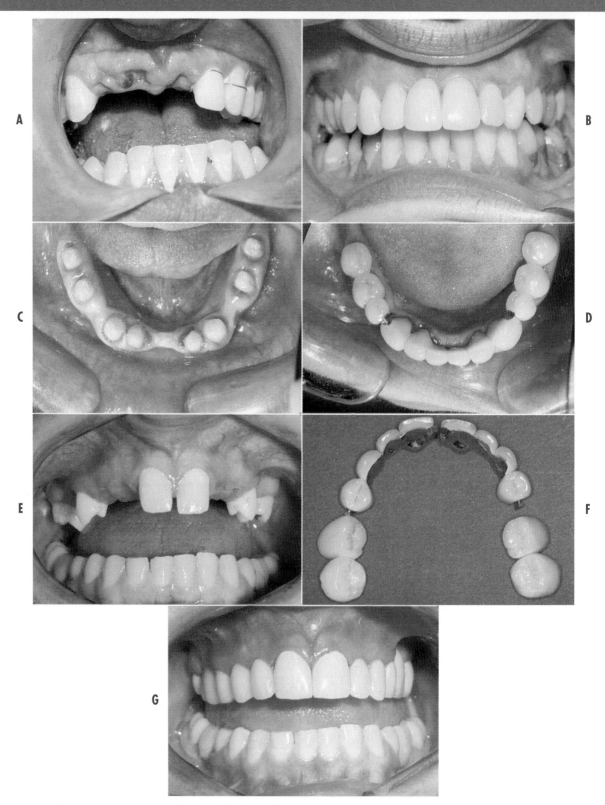

FIG. 16.21   Multiple-unit fixed prostheses (bridges) made of porcelain fused to metal, are strong, beautiful, and long lasting. But, they are expensive. **A** to **D,** Accident patient before and after. **E** to **G,** Fixed prostheses in a person with permanent teeth missing from birth. You can't find better replacements for any missing body part!

loaded. Patients need to "favor" the bridged areas slightly to avoid overloading and potentially loosening or damaging the prostheses.

C. **Risks:** Extra load on the supporting teeth of the bridge can weaken, break, or cause pulp death in these abutments (teeth). The crowns (caps) that connect to the supporting abutments can come loose, potentially causing dental caries (decay) on the supporting teeth. Pieces of porcelain or resin (plastic) can break away from a part of the bridge, causing the need for repair or replacement.

D. **Alternatives:** Removable partial dentures are the most common alternatives (p. 162), but implants with crowns (caps) and/or fixed prostheses placed over them (p. 152), or Maryland bridges are also acceptable (p. 152).

E. **Cost:** The cost of a fixed prosthesis relates to the number of teeth missing. A bridge replacing one tooth usually requires placement of crowns (caps) on one tooth on each side of the space. The replacement of one tooth costs the same amount for three crowns (caps). Removable prostheses or Maryland bridges are less expensive (p. 152). Fixed prostheses are among the most expensive treatments in dentistry, but patient acceptance and satisfaction is very positive. Nearly all patients say that the treatment result justifies the cost.

F. **Result of Nontreatment (see Fig. 16.5):** When one or several missing teeth are not replaced, the surrounding teeth collapse toward the space, and the opposing teeth grow (extrude) into the space. The resultant collapsed bite gradually worsens, and both appearance and function are compromised.

7. Fixed Prosthesis, Cantilever

(FIG. 16.22). In a few locations in the mouth, a fixed prosthesis may be constructed that connects to one or more teeth on only one end of

the missing tooth space, replacing one or more missing teeth. The most common situation is when one front tooth adjacent to the two center teeth (lateral incisor) is missing. The canine (eye) tooth is trimmed down, and a crown (cap) is cemented onto the canine tooth that replaces the lateral incisor also. In some cases these fixed prostheses are the treatment of choice.

A. **Advantages:** Only one tooth is prepared (trimmed down) instead of two, and the cost is lower.

B. **Disadvantages:** The patient must exercise some care to avoid chewing extremely hard foods on the replacement tooth.

C. **Risks:** Infrequently, there is unplanned movement of the nonprepared tooth adjacent to the missing tooth space. In such cases, an unsightly small space or altered tooth alignment may occur. Cantilever prostheses are not as strong

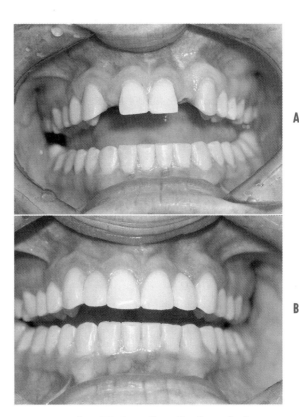

A

B

FIG. 16.22 **A and B,** A cantilever fixed prosthesis replaces a missing tooth but only attaches to one natural tooth. The one shown replaces the lateral incisors and attaches to the canines (eye teeth). These are excellent, long-lasting restorations.

as bridges with abutments on both sides of the missing tooth space.

D. **Alternatives:** A fixed prosthesis connected to teeth on both sides of the space (p. 152), a removable partial denture (p. 162), implants and crown(s) (cap[s]) (p. 152), or Maryland bridges (p. 152) are also acceptable.

E. **Cost:** This alternative is less expensive than a fixed prosthesis connected to teeth on both sides of the space, but it is more expensive than a removable partial denture. (See costs of fixed prosthesis [p. 151].)

F. **Result of Nontreatment:** Tooth movement of all surrounding and opposing teeth will take place, compromising function and appearance (see Fig. 16.5).

8. Fixed Prosthesis, Maryland Bridge

(FIG. 16.23). Occasionally, missing teeth may be replaced conservatively by acid etching the enamel of the teeth adjacent to the space, making microscopic irregularities on the enamel surface. These irregularities afford retention and bonding. Very thin pieces of metal are bonded with resin (plastic) to the back surfaces of the acid-etched (roughened) tooth enamel surfaces. These pieces of metal hold a beautiful artificial tooth in place.

A. **Advantages:** Adjacent teeth are not trimmed down as much as for traditional fixed prostheses, and the cost is somewhat lower.

B. **Disadvantages:** Many of these prostheses are not as pleasing in appearance as conventional porcelain-fused-to-metal (PFM) fixed prostheses because the gray color of the metal may show through the tooth.

C. **Risks:** A blow to the face or chewing on hard or sticky substances can loosen the Maryland bridge from the supporting teeth.

D. **Alternatives:** Cantilever fixed prostheses (p. 151), traditional fixed prostheses (p. 149), implant(s) and crowns (caps) (p. 152), and removable partial dentures (p. 162) are acceptable alternatives.

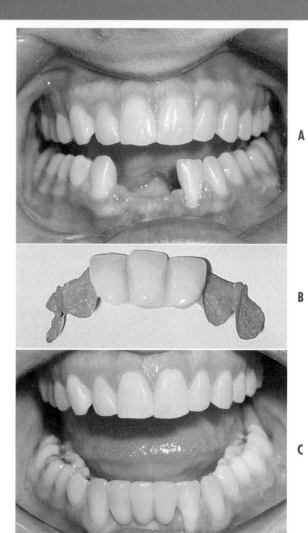

FIG. 16.23   A, These three lower missing teeth are replaced with a Maryland bridge, which is a very conservative treatment. In this case, two teeth on each side of the space were etched with acid (roughened), and the prosthesis shown in **B** was attached with resin (plastic) cement to the natural teeth **(C).**

E. **Cost:** Maryland bridges usually cost less than traditional fixed prostheses and more than removable prostheses.

F. **Result of Nontreatment:** Tooth movement of all surrounding and opposing teeth will take place, compromising function and appearance.

9. Crowns (Caps) or Fixed Prostheses Placed Over Implants

(FIG. 16.24). In some situations a dental implant(s) can be placed in the site of the missing tooth (teeth), and bridges or crowns

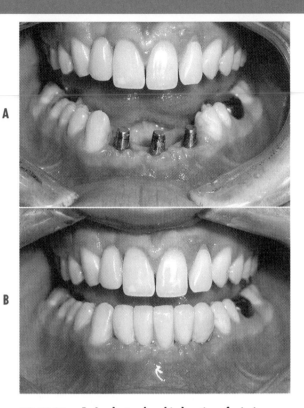

FIG. 16.24 **A,** Implants placed in location of missing teeth on lower arch. **B,** Fixed bridge cemented over implants to replace missing teeth.

(caps) can be placed on the implants replacing the missing teeth. This is an excellent alternative when it is possible, but not all dentists perform these procedures, and referral to a periodontist, oral surgeon, and/or prosthodontist may be necessary. Refer to the chapter on implants (p. 61) for more information.

A. **Advantages:** Surrounding natural teeth may not be affected. The prostheses look and feel like normal teeth.

B. **Disadvantages:** The cost of the implant(s) is significant, and implants require a healing period of 4 to 6 months before the crowns (caps) or bridges can be placed.

C. **Risks:** Occasionally the implants fail, and when this occurs, the crowns (caps) or bridges fail also, and other types of tooth replacements must be made.

D. **Alternatives:** Cantilever fixed prostheses (p. 151), traditional fixed prostheses (p. 149), and removable partial den-

tures (p. 162) are acceptable alternatives for crowns (caps) or bridges over implants.

E. **Cost:** There is one cost for the implants, and another for the crowns (caps) or bridges. An average fee for a single implant is about the cost of one and a half to two crowns (caps). Therefore, the cost of replacing teeth with crowns (caps) or bridges over implants is high. Removable partial dentures cost less but have disadvantages (p. 162).

F. **Result of Nontreatment:** Tooth movement of all surrounding and opposing teeth will take place, compromising function and appearance.

10. Repair of Fixed Prosthesis (Bridge or Crown [Cap])

The cost of a fixed prosthesis or crown (cap) is high, and it is often desirable to repair these restorations if possible. How do crowns (caps) or fixed prostheses fail? Numerous types of failure occur, including the following:

- The crown (cap) loosens from the underlying tooth. If this restoration is a single crown (cap) and dental decay is not a problem, the crown (cap) can usually be recemented onto the remaining tooth preparation. If the loose crown (cap) is a portion of a fixed prosthesis and only one end of the prosthesis is loose, it may not be salvageable. The underlying tooth structure on the loose end of the bridge may be decayed, and the crown (cap) on the other end of the bridge may be attached too tightly to be removed. In such a case, remaking the fixed prosthesis is the best option.

- Dental caries (decay) can occur at the junction of the tooth and the crown (cap) or bridge. If this condition is observed at an early stage, repair is often simple, but if allowed to progress, simple repair may be impossible.

- A piece of the tooth-colored part of the fixed prosthesis (porcelain) can break away, leaving metal exposed underneath. Repair of this condition may range from simple to impossible. Various repair materials and techniques are used, ranging from plastic attached to the broken part of the crown (cap) or bridge to a new "over crown" (cap) cemented over one or more of the broken teeth on the fixed prosthesis.

- A hole can be worn in the chewing surface of the crown (cap) or fixed prosthesis. Usually this condition can be repaired easily with a simple restoration (filling).
- The pulp (nerve) in the tooth supporting a crown (cap) or part of a fixed prosthesis dies. This condition is usually repaired relatively easily by making a small hole in the chewing surface of the crown (cap) or fixed prosthesis, completing endodontics (root canal therapy) through the hole, placing a strengthening post, and filling the hole.

A. **Advantages of Repairing a Fixed Prosthesis or Crown (Cap):** The major reason for repair instead of replacement is significantly lower cost. Also, less time is required for the patient to accommodate to a repair than to a new crown (cap) or fixed prosthesis.

B. **Disadvantages:** Simple repairs have few or no disadvantages, and they are the treatment of choice when possible. More complex repairs often compromise the strength or appearance of the crown (cap) or fixed prosthesis, thereby reducing long-term acceptability. Money spent on a complex repair may be wasted if the crown (cap) or fixed prosthesis requires redoing soon after the repair.

C. **Risks:** Simple repairs have few or no risks, but complex repairs are often very difficult for the practitioner and may not allow adequate visual observation of the situation. Failure may occur soon.

D. **Alternatives:** Remaking the crown (cap) or fixed prosthesis is usually the most adequate alternative. In the case of complex repair need, this is usually stronger and better in appearance.

E. **Cost:** The major motivation for repair is less cost than redoing the procedure. Cost of a repair may range from the relatively low fee of a simple filling to more than half the cost of a new crown (cap) or fixed prosthesis.

F. **Result of Nontreatment:** If a crown (cap) or fixed prosthesis (fixed bridge) is loose and treatment is not accomplished, significant degeneration will continue. If dental caries (decay) is present and is not repaired, destruction of the tooth will occur eventually. If a piece of tooth-colored material is broken away from the crown (cap) or fixed prosthesis, there is usually no physiological danger to leaving the defect, and it is only disagreeable in appearance. If a dead or dying pulp (nerve) is left under a crown (cap) or fixed prosthesis, bone destruction and/or pain will continue until you are forced to treat the condition.

SUMMARY

Fixed prosthodontics usually provides an excellent esthetic result, and it is one of the most accepted, long term, and potentially satisfying therapies of all areas in dentistry. Single or multiple broken-down teeth, or missing teeth, can be repaired or replaced very acceptably using currently available high-quality techniques and materials. Competent general practitioners or prosthodontists must be found for this service, and you should expect the treatment to be significantly more expensive than normal restorations (fillings).

CHAPTER 17

Prosthodontics, Removable
Dentures Replacing All or Some Teeth

Among the most well known but least desired areas of dentistry is removable prosthodontics. However, well-made and fitted artificial dentures can be relatively satisfactory replacements for teeth and surrounding bone and soft tissue for a predictable period. Unknown to many persons is the fact that the jawbones and gum tissues shrink a known amount when teeth are removed, and even more upsetting is that shrinkage continues to occur throughout the remainder of the person's life. Acceptance of this fact is a major decision for a person considering tooth removal. Frustration with the maintenance of natural teeth can lead a person to think that tooth removal is an easy solution. However, tooth removal usually substitutes other problems for the one you are trying to avoid. Usually, but not always, retention of natural teeth is the best decision. Having your teeth removed can be compared to having an arm amputated. You can get a new artificial arm, but it will never function as well as the original arm. If you have lost some or all of your natural teeth, you should find a general dentist whose practice includes removable prosthodontics or a prosthodontist for acceptable treatment.

WHAT YOU SEE OR FEEL

Conditions, Signs, or Symptoms Related to Removable Prosthodontics

Implants are among the best ways to replace missing teeth, and Chapter 10 on implant dentistry should be read in addition to this chapter.

1. One or More Teeth Missing

(FIG. 17.1). The signs and symptoms of one or more teeth missing are described in the section on fixed prosthodontics. *Please refer to that information about what you see or feel* (p. 140). Most persons prefer to have one of the fixed prosthodontic options (bridge attached into mouth) when one or many teeth are missing, but for financial or other reasons removable prosthodontic options may be best. All of the treatment alternatives follow, some of which are removable prostheses:

A. Fixed prosthesis (traditional bridge involving at least one tooth on each side of space as abutment teeth) (p. 149)

B. Fixed prosthesis (Maryland bridge) (less prepared [trimmed] teeth on each side of the space, with conservative bridge holding a false tooth, usually leaving the front portion of the abutment teeth intact) (p. 152)

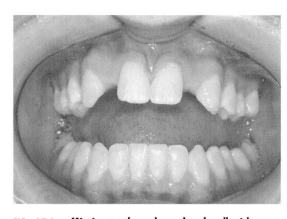

FIG. 17.1 **Missing teeth can be replaced well with either fixed or removable prostheses (dentures); most people prefer fixed.**

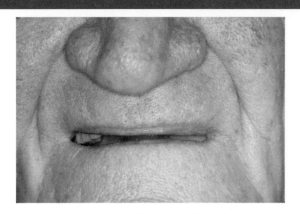

FIG. 17.2　Removal of all natural teeth produces a sunken, aged look.

C. Cantilever fixed prosthesis (traditional bridge involving one or more teeth on one side of space only as abutments) (p. 151)

D. Removable partial denture (all plastic) (p. 162)

E. Removable partial denture (traditional metal and plastic) (p. 162)

F. Removable partial denture, precision or semi-precision (plastic and metal fitted to crowns [caps]) (p. 162)

G. Implant(s) with crown(s) (caps) or prosthesis fixed on top to replace teeth (p. 72)

H. Implant(s) with removable partial denture placed on top of them (p. 70)

2. All Teeth Missing in Upper and/or Lower Jaw(s)

(FIG. 17.2). This unfortunate condition occurs less frequently now than in past decades, but it is still relatively common. Your treatment alternatives are the following:

A. Removable complete denture(s) (p. 163)

B. Implants with fixed prosthesis on top of them to replace teeth (p. 69)

C. Implants with removable denture(s) placed on top of them (p. 66)

3. All Teeth in Upper and/or Lower Arch Degenerated to the Extent That They Must Be Removed

Numerous conditions cause this situation, including dental caries (decay), gum and bone disease (periodontal disease), accidents, congenital deformities or other abnormalities, cancer requiring radiation and/or chemotherapy, or other conditions. When all of the teeth must be removed, some decisions must be made as to whether the teeth should be:

1. Removed all at once and the bone and gums allowed to heal before placing the denture(s) later. Usually this treatment is not one of the options, because the person must be toothless for several weeks before the denture(s) can be placed.

2. Removed partially (back teeth first), letting those areas heal without any replacements, and then, on the next appointment, removing the remaining front teeth and placing denture(s) to replace all teeth. This treatment is called a staged immediate denture. The person is never completely toothless **(see Fig. 17-16).**

3. Removed completely on one day, and during the same appointment, denture(s) placed to replace all of the teeth. This is a complete immediate denture. All the remaining degenerate natural teeth are left in the mouth until placement of the denture(s). Most people elect the latter two options because the new denture(s) serve as a type of bandage to help the bone and gums to heal.

4. Conditions Involved With Partial or Complete Denture(s)

Patient dissatisfaction with removable dentures is known to be one of the highest of any area of dentistry. The facts are that natural teeth are meant to remain in the mouth, and that artificial removable dentures replace natural teeth to only a small portion of their original effectiveness. Also, we all have varying abilities to tolerate the many challenges of removable complete dentures. Some of the following conditions can be corrected easily, whereas others may not have simple solutions. The conditions listed are followed by alternative solutions described in the next section of this chapter, What Your Prosthodontist or General Dentist Can Do.

A. My dentures collect food under them.
SOLUTION: Reline (p. 160), rebase

(p. 161), or make new dentures (p. 163).

B. My denture bases (pink portion) are discolored. SOLUTION: Clean and polish denture (p. 157), rebase (p. 161), or make new dentures (p. 163).

C. The denture teeth are discolored. SOLUTION: Clean and polish denture (p. 157), replace teeth (p. 160), or make new denture (p. 163).

D. I can't chew well. SOLUTION: Make new denture (p. 163) or repair denture by sharpening existing teeth (p. 160).

E. My gums have sore spots. SOLUTION: Adjust denture (p. 158), reline (p. 160), rebase (p. 161), or make new denture (p. 163).

F. My gums hurt when I chew. SOLUTION: Adjust denture (p. 158), reline (p. 160), rebase (p. 161), or make new denture (p. 163).

G. I bite my cheeks or tongue. SOLUTION: Repair denture by recontouring teeth (p. 160), or make new denture (p. 163).

H. The dentures won't stay in place. SOLUTION: Reline (p. 160), rebase (p. 161), or make new dentures (p. 163).

I. The dentures have missing or broken teeth. SOLUTION: Repair denture by replacing teeth (p. 160), or make new denture (p. 163).

J. The dentures are broken. SOLUTION: Repair (p. 160), or make new dentures (p. 163).

K. My nose and my chin are too close together when I bite down with the dentures in place. Solution: Make new dentures (p. 163).

L. My dentures have worn the teeth or crowns on my opposing jaw. SOLUTION: Make new dentures using less abrasive denture teeth (p. 160) and repair natural teeth, repair, or make new crowns (caps) (p. 147).

M. My dentures have a poor bite. SOLUTION: Repair dentures by selective grinding or sharpening teeth (p. 161), or make new dentures (p. 163).

N. My removable partial dentures cause pain in the supporting natural teeth when I chew. SOLUTION: Adjust retaining clasps of removable partial denture (p. 158), or make new partial denture (p. 162).

O. The clasps (retaining wires) on my partial denture show too much. SOLUTION: Make new partial denture (p. 162).

P. The supporting teeth for my removable partial denture are loose. SOLUTION: Treat supporting teeth if necessary, and repair or make new removable partial dentures (p. 162).

Q. A supporting tooth for my removable partial denture is broken or decayed. SOLUTION: Repair supporting tooth and retrofit partial denture to repaired tooth (p. 159).

R. My dentures are too tight. SOLUTION: Adjust dentures (p. 158).

WHAT YOUR PROSTHODONTIST OR GENERAL DENTIST CAN DO

Treatment Available

Several types of treatment are available in the area of removable prosthodontics. Most general dentists accomplish some removable prosthodontic procedures, but if your condition is especially complex, or if you have had difficulty with previous prosthodontic treatment, then you may want to seek the services of a prosthodontist (a dentist specially educated in prosthodontics) (p. 15).

1. Repairing Previous Removable Partial or Complete Prosthesis (Denture)

Repair may be a choice, but it will probably be only a temporary remedy that will require more comprehensive therapy later. Consult your dentist to determine the desirability or feasibility of repairing your current prosthesis (denture). The following are relatively simple, common maintenance or repair procedures for dentures that may satisfy your needs without requiring a new denture:

i. *Cleaning and polishing* (FIG. 17.3): Stains, food, tartar, and accumulation of

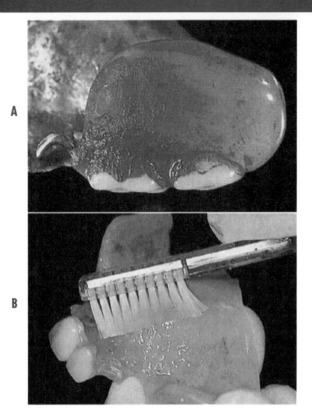

FIG. 17.3 **A,** Denture needs a thorough cleaning by the dentist; this denture has been stained with a red dye. **B,** Cleaning by a patient, which will prevent gross accumulation of debris but cannot remove severe deposits. (From Davenport JC et al: *A clinical guide to removable partial dentures,* London, 2001, Macmillan.)

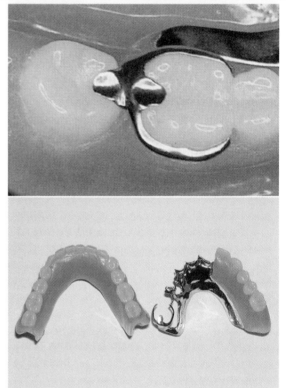

FIG. 17.4 **A,** Metallic clasps hold removable partial dentures in place. **B,** Removable partial dentures are held in by metallic clasps *(right),* whereas complete dentures fit on the gums only *(left).* (From Davenport JC et al: *A clinical guide to removable partial denture design,* London, in press, Macmillan.)

dental plaque can make a denture disagreeable in appearance and uncomfortable. Dentures need to be cleaned and polished often to remove these accumulations. This procedure is simple, fast, effective, and inexpensive.

ii. *Adjusting base or other portion of the denture:* The most common need in removable prosthodontics is adjustment of the base of the denture (the portion that sits on the gums). Even a slight amount of extra denture length, and the associated pressure on the gums and bone, can cause mild to severe pain for the denture wearer and dissatisfaction with the denture. Usually these sore spots are located on the denture base and are found by using pressure pastes inside the denture while moderate biting pressure is placed on the denture by the wearer.

Removal of the pressure spot in the denture provides almost instant relief. Denture wearers who are in good health should have no difficulty having dentists locate and treat denture sore spots. Chronic sore spots that do not respond to repeated denture adjustments may require other treatment, such as relining or rebasing the denture or making a new one.

iii. *Adjusting retentive metal clasps (wirelike portions) of a removable partial denture* (FIG. 17.4): Partial dentures usually become looser as they are worn for a period of months or years. As they loosen, they are often difficult to keep in the mouth, which is annoying, and food tends to collect under them. Your dentist can accomplish adjustment of the retentive clasps to make them tighter. This procedure

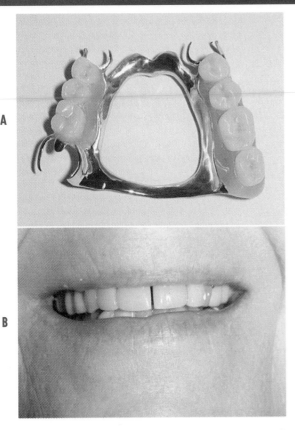

FIG. 17.5 **A,** Three teeth support the removable partial denture. If one of the abutment teeth breaks, it can be removed and will still fit the partial. **B,** Note that the partial denture in place does not show metal.

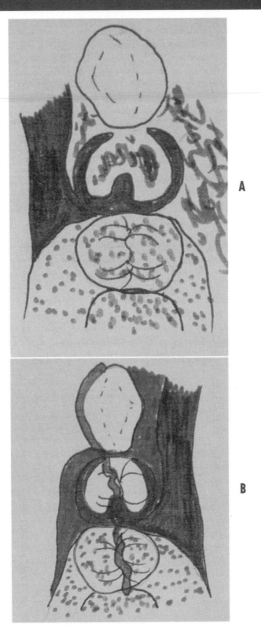

FIG. 17.6 Replacement of a removed natural tooth that supported a removable partial denture **(A)** is possible by adding an artificial tooth to the denture, along with a new clasp **(B).**

may look simple to you, but even experienced dentists find it threatening, since the clasps are often brittle and can be broken relatively easily. Overtightening can cause pain in the supporting teeth. Adjustment should be accomplished when needed, but it should not be overdone.

iv. *Repairing a tooth that supports removable partial denture* **(FIG. 17.5):** An abutment tooth that is painful or broken cannot support a partial denture well. Repair of that tooth may be very simple or complex. It can require something as simple as a small restoration (filling) (p. 170), or as complex as an endodontic procedure (root canal) (p. 40) followed by a new crown (cap) (p. 147) that is fitted to the already existing partial denture. Occasionally a supporting tooth for the partial denture must be removed because

of some nonrepairable situation. In such a case, new retentive clasps (wires) may be fitted to the existing partial denture to salvage it for additional use **(FIG. 17.6).** Your dentist can tell you about the complexity of repair for a partial denture (supporting tooth). Infrequently, if supporting tooth removal is required, a new partial denture or other treatment must be accomplished.

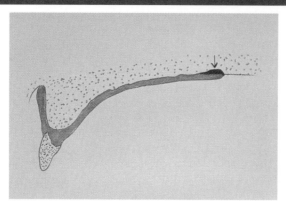

FIG. 17.7 Arrow shows area of repair to the denture, providing better seal and retention of the denture (schematic cross section drawing).

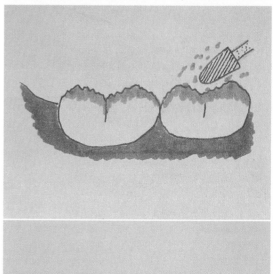
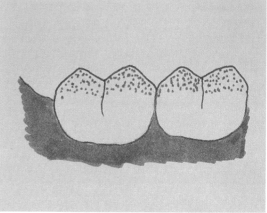

FIG. 17.8 Roughening the surface of old plastic denture teeth **(A)** may allow rebuilding of the teeth with new plastic **(B)**.

v. *Repairing cracked, broken, or ill-fitting complete or partial denture:* If a denture is cracked or broken, undue stress usually has been placed on it, or the fracture has occurred accidentally. Dentures that crack while chewing may be subjected to too much stress, or may require more thickness or reinforcement during construction. The repair of such stressed dentures may not be the preferred treatment, since repair usually weakens the original denture. Occasionally, additions to dentures are required for improvement of retention **(FIG. 17.7)**. Consult with your dentist on such conditions. Dentures that have been broken accidentally or need additions can usually be repaired easily, successfully, and relatively inexpensively.

vi. *Replacing tooth (teeth) on a removable partial or complete denture:* This type of denture problem is a simple one that requires minimal time and cost. If other aspects of the denture are acceptable, there is usually no reason to do anything other than replace the missing tooth (teeth).

vii. *Reshaping or reforming denture teeth on a removable partial or complete denture* **(FIG. 17.8)**: Patients complain occasionally about biting their lips, cheeks, or tongue. Sometimes this problem is difficult to overcome. Often it is related only to past chewing habits that wear the teeth into a flat plane, thus pinching and biting the lips, cheeks, or tongue. Reshaping the teeth to eliminate flat surfaces usually corrects this annoying and painful problem. Denture teeth shaped with points, grooves, and valleys can help make chewing more efficient also.

viii. *Relining removable partial or complete dentures* **(FIG. 17.9)**: Dentures that have been worn for months to years may not have adequate tight adaptation to the mouth soft tissues because these tissues have shrunk. This is a continuing process that is normal and should be expected. Relining a denture means that the internal portion of the denture is relieved (ground out)

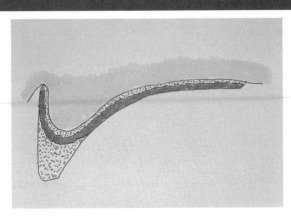

FIG. 17.9 **Relining dentures should be expected every few years because of shrinkage of oral soft tissue and bone (schematic cross section drawing).**

by the dentist, an impression is made inside the denture, and the internal surface of the denture is replaced with new plastic material that is the same color as the original pink denture base.

This procedure may be accomplished either in one appointment while you wait in the office, or in two appointments—one to make the impression and another one to place the denture. This second type of reline (laboratory reline) is usually the preferred type because of better fit; it is also more expensive than the in-office type, and it requires you to be without the denture for up to 24 hours.

Another variable in denture relines is the availability of both hard and soft relining material. Some clinical situations require soft reline material, but most denture relines may be accomplished well with hard material similar to the original denture base. If soft relines are placed in the denture, they provide a cushion for the biting forces and are then usually more comfortable than hard denture relines. However, soft relining material lasts only a few months to a few years.

ix. *Rebasing removable partial or complete dentures:* Frequently, when con-

sidering relining or rebasing dentures, the teeth (tooth-colored portions), the occlusion (bite), and the tooth positioning are still acceptable. Only the fit, positioning, and extension of the denture bases are unacceptable. In such cases, a rebase of the denture may be suggested. In this situation, all of the pink material of the denture is replaced, compared with denture relining, in which only the internal portion of the denture is lined. Rebasing a denture is more expensive than relining the same denture, but it is still less expensive than making a new denture. A properly rebased denture can look and feel like a new one. Rebased dentures may have soft or hard internal portions, with a shorter longevity for the soft liner.

A. **Advantages of Repairing Previous Removable Partial or Complete Prosthesis:** If the prosthesis is basically satisfactory to you and is only broken, missing some teeth, cracked, or ill-fitting, repairing it is less of a physiological or psychological shock than remaking the denture. The cost to repair the denture is also less than to remake it.

B. **Disadvantages:** Only infrequently can repair of a denture make it better than it was before it needed repair, whereas making a new denture can potentially make a more acceptable prosthesis in both appearance and function. Sometimes, repaired dentures are weaker than the original denture. Your dentist will be able to advise you concerning the desirability of repairing versus remaking your denture.

C. **Risks:** Repairing an existing denture is similar to placing a new sole on a shoe—you still have part of the old shoe remaining, with unknown internal defects and longevity. Nevertheless, repair of existing dentures is often a wise decision.

D. **Alternatives:** Only one alternative is present if change is desired—making a new denture.

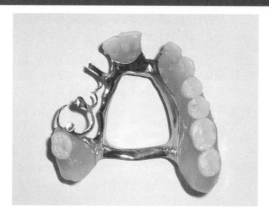

FIG. 17.10 **Removable partial denture replacing several upper teeth.**

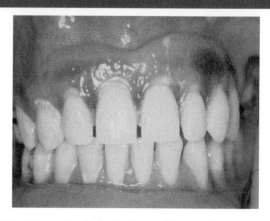

FIG. 17.11 **An all-plastic denture blends with the oral environment well, but it does not have the same strength or support as a denture reinforced with metal.** (From Davenport JC et al: *A clinical guide to removable partial dentures*, London, 2001, Macmillan.)

E. **Cost:** You should expect a relatively low cost for these services compared with the cost of making a new denture. Small repairs or replacement of missing teeth is inexpensive, whereas relining a denture is moderate in cost, and rebasing a denture is the most expensive of the repair procedures.

F. **Result of Nontreatment:** Minor need for repair can be tolerated without significant handicap, whereas broken or ill-fitting dentures require immediate attention. Avoiding a reline or rebase when a denture is ill fitting can cause significant damage to the gums and remaining bone support.

2. Removable Partial Denture

(FIG. 17.10). Removable partial dentures, replacing teeth and missing gum tissue, can be functional and highly pleasing in appearance, or they can be unacceptable, depending on the patient's clinical situation. These prostheses must be taken out of the mouth daily for cleaning. They usually attach to the remaining natural teeth for retention, and the clasps (wires) holding them in place may or may not be acceptable in appearance, depending on the situation. There are three major types of removable partial dentures:

   i. All plastic, no metal: tooth-colored teeth, with a gum-colored, all-plastic base **(FIG. 17.11)**

   ii. Conventional removable partial denture: tooth-colored teeth and gum-colored plastic base, with metal framework and clasps resting on and gaining support from remaining teeth **(FIG. 17.12)**

   iii. Semi-precision or precision removable partial denture **(FIG. 17.13):** tooth-colored teeth and gum-colored plastic base supported by metal framework and precision-fitted attachments into crowns (caps) on remaining teeth

A. **Advantages:** All-plastic and conventional partial dentures replace missing teeth in the easiest and least expensive way. They usually do not require alteration of remaining natural teeth. Precision or semi-precision partial dentures can be highly functional and pleasing in appearance.

B. **Disadvantages:** Removable partial dentures must be removed several times per day for cleaning. Food collects under them occasionally, and they may be broken while out of the mouth. Generally, as judged by patients, removable partial dentures are much less successful than fixed partial dentures. Also, certain designs may be less pleasing in appearance than desired.

C. **Risks:** Supporting teeth can be broken, loosened, or weakened. Partial dentures may be lost occasionally. A few patients have swallowed small remov-

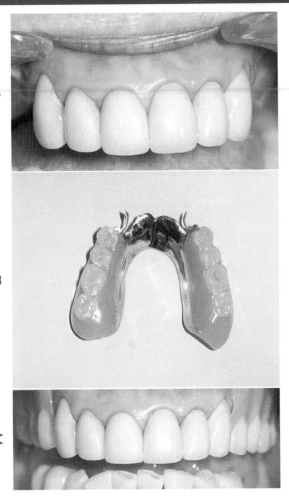

FIG. 17.12 **A,** Upper arch with all back teeth missing. **B,** Removable partial denture. **C,** Denture in place.

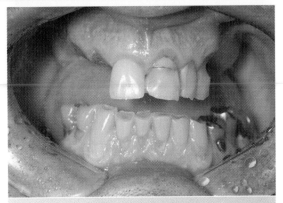

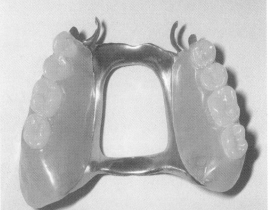

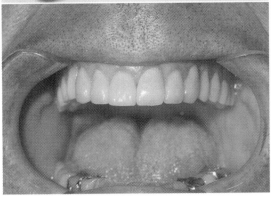

FIG. 17.13 **A,** Patient requiring upper rehabilitation. **B,** Semi-precision removable partial denture. **C,** Six front crowns (caps) and removable partial denture in place.

able partial dentures, causing significant problems.

D. **Cost:** All-plastic partial dentures are inexpensive, while conventional partials are intermediate in cost, and semi-precision and precision removable partials are expensive (often about the cost of fixed partial dentures).

E. **Alternatives:** Fixed partial dentures (p. 152), crowns (caps) over implants (p. 72), or removable partial dentures over implants (p. 70) can be made.

F. **Result of Nontreatment:** Persons who elect not to replace missing teeth continue to have an abnormal appearance and smile, have difficulty chewing in direct relation to the number of teeth that are missing, and experience movement of teeth over a period of time and resulting malocclusion (poor bite).

3. Removable Complete Dentures

(FIG. 17.14). Millions of people wear complete dentures because their natural teeth have been lost for various reasons. The functional success, comfort, and appearance of these dentures vary enormously. Many people are satisfied with their artificial dentures, but most patients have occasional to constant discomfort, reduced chewing efficiency compared with natural teeth, and some facial collapse. Upper dentures are tolerated much better than lower dentures. Total removal of

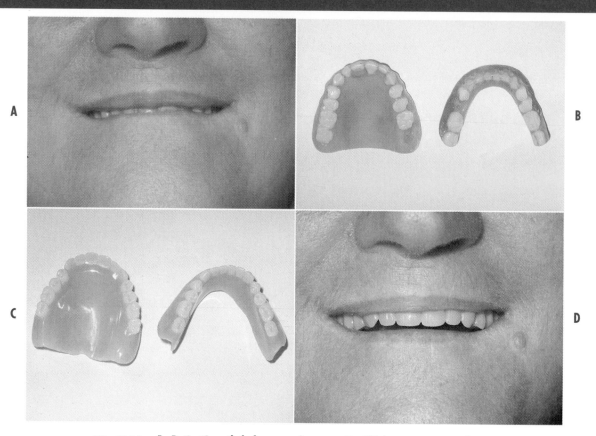

FIG. 17.14 **A,** Patient's smile before new dentures. **B,** Old dentures, worn and discolored. **C,** New dentures. **D,** Patient's smile with new dentures.

teeth is a shock to the body and leaves the chewing system handicapped in most situations. The degree of handicap relates directly to the type and quality of the prosthesis (denture) made. Quality of complete denture prostheses varies significantly, and it is often related to fee. Additionally, the dentist and technician making the denture relate to its acceptability. Many general dentists do a fine job with standard uncomplicated dentures, but if you have had significant problems with your denture in the past, or you know that you have a difficult case, you may want to seek the services of a prosthodontist (p. 15).

Construction of removable complete dentures usually requires several nonobjectionable appointments, during which the dentist determines the optimal function for your specific situation, as well as the most acceptable appearance for your facial and dental areas.

A. **Advantages:** Removable complete dentures are better than no teeth at all, restoring at least some of the original preextraction form and function of nat-

ural teeth. They can be cleaned outside the mouth. Repair of natural teeth has been eliminated by the extractions, but constantly changing soft and hard oral tissues require that the artificial dentures and your remaining mouth tissue have continued observation and therapy.

B. **Disadvantages:** Dentures provide only some of the original chewing efficiency and beauty of natural teeth. The bone of the jaws and gum tissues continue to shrink and change **(FIG. 17.15)** for the duration of your life, requiring relining (p. 160), rebasing (p. 161), or remaking of the denture periodically. Although many persons wear the same set of dentures for many years, a dentist easily observes the damage to the denture-wearer's jawbone caused by the ill-fitting denture. Dentures should be refitted every few years by relining or rebasing, and new dentures should be made every 5 to 10 years because of the significant oral shrinkage that is always present.

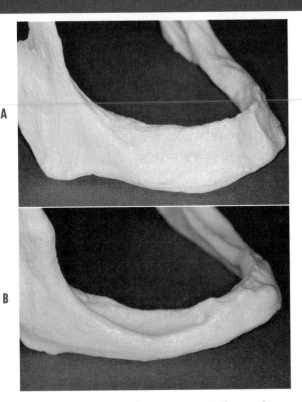

FIG. 17.15   **A,** Shape of lower jaw soon after teeth have been removed. **B,** Shrinkage of lower jaw several years later.

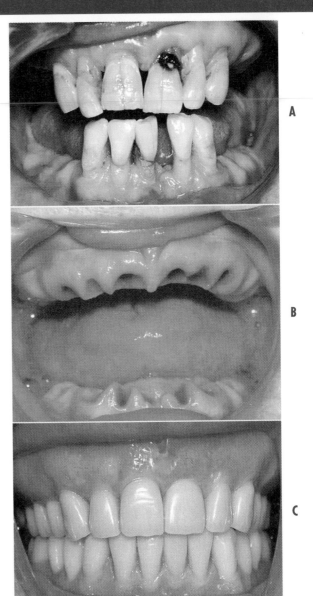

FIG. 17.16   **A,** Person requiring removal of all teeth; back teeth had been removed previously. **B,** Day of tooth removal. **C,** Immediate placement of dentures on day of tooth removal.

C. **Risks:** Shrinkage of oral tissues continues throughout life when natural teeth are not present. If dentures are not refitted as described above, damage to the mouth can occur, ranging from chronic sore spots to oral cancer.

D. **Cost:** Fees for artificial dentures range from low to high. Generally, cost relates directly to denture quality and its ability to serve with comfort. Don't select a dentist based on lower cost; usually you will pay for that decision eventually.

E. **Alternatives:** Only two alternatives are possible. Placement of several implants followed by a fixed denture provides function nearly as acceptable as that of natural teeth (p. 69). The other alternative is placement of at least two implants followed by a removable denture attached to the implants. This treatment significantly improves the satisfaction enjoyed by complete-denture wearers.

F. **Result of Nontreatment:** Failure to wear complete dentures results in impaired chewing and nutrition, intestinal distress, abnormal aged facial appearance, altered speech, and overall lowered self-esteem.

4. Removable Immediate Complete Denture
(FIG. 17.16). Immediate dentures were previously discussed in this chapter (p. 156). When teeth and/or supporting oral structures have degenerated to the extent that complete dentures must be considered, most people

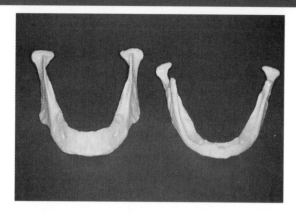

FIG. 17.17   Note shrinkage of lower jawbone on right, which cannot be avoided after teeth are removed.

elect to have the natural teeth removed and the dentures placed on the same appointment. All of the teeth may be removed on the day the immediate dentures are placed, or some teeth in the back portion of the mouth (molars and premolars) may be removed on one day, allowing healing for about 6 weeks before the front teeth are removed and the dentures placed during the second appointment on another day. After initial healing of the jawbones and gums, the same slow shrinkage of these structures continues to occur throughout life, as described in the section on removable complete dentures (p. 163) (FIG. 17.17). When a removable partial denture is indicated and some teeth must be extracted, the removable partial denture may be made also as an immediate partial denture.

A. **Advantages:** There is no time when you do not have teeth. You either have your own teeth or the removable complete immediate denture. The immediate denture serves as a splint for the healing oral tissues, thereby decreasing the discomfort during the healing process.

B. **Disadvantages:** The change from natural teeth to dentures in one day is a shock. Patients report that chewing, speech, and overall awareness of teeth change significantly, requiring a period of psychological and physical adjustment to the new situation. The immediate denture must be relined (p. 160) about 6 weeks or more after removal of the teeth to fit the denture to the initially healed gums. This requires the patient to be without teeth for anywhere from 8 to 24 hours.

C. **Risks:** In addition to the risks described under removable complete dentures (p. 163), only the normal surgical risks are involved with immediate dentures. Most people feel that having their dentures constructed on an immediate basis is far better than having their teeth removed, staying toothless for 6 or more weeks, and having a removable complete denture made at that time.

D. **Alternatives:** Teeth may be removed and the tissues allowed to heal for 6 weeks before placing the dentures. (Removable complete denture, p. 163) Teeth may be removed and implants placed, thereby allowing a fixed (p. 69) or removable (p. 66) implant prosthesis to be made.

E. **Cost:** The cost of this therapy is based on the following factors: 1) surgical removal of the teeth, 2) making the denture, and 3) relining the denture after the oral tissues have healed. The overall cost of this therapy is moderate to high for most situations.

F. **Result of Nontreatment:** If your teeth need to be removed and you do not do so, infection, pain, continued discomfort, reduced function, and unpleasant appearance will gradually occur. These factors will force you to have the teeth removed eventually.

SUMMARY

Removable prosthodontics, which usually involves removal of some or all of the natural teeth and replacement with dentures, is one of the most feared treatments for most patients. It is also among the least acceptable of all areas of dentistry. However, if it must be done, well-constructed and properly fitted removable partial or complete dentures can serve you well, with your cooperation.

CHAPTER 18

Restorative or Operative Dentistry
Fillings for Teeth

The most common and well known treatment accomplished in the general dentist's office is filling or restoring teeth. Although restoration (filling) of teeth involves a significant amount of time in many general practices, you are learning from this book that dentists do far more than restore teeth. However, dental caries (decay) is still common in most parts of the world, and the routine restoration of teeth continues to be a significant part of dentistry. In developing countries, dental caries among children is high. Less dental caries is present in children in developed countries, where the disease has shifted to the other end of life in the now long-lived mature population. Dental caries has long been the most prevalent of all oral diseases, and you probably have some restorations (fillings) in your teeth. Chapter 19 tells you how to prevent this common disease relatively easily.

Dental caries usually develops in the grooves found on the chewing surfaces of the teeth or between the teeth, but the breakdown of tooth surfaces can occur in any location on teeth where food debris is left routinely (FIG. 18.1). Dental caries is not painful at first, but when pain is present while eating cold foods, sugar, or other stimulation, the degenerative process has progressed to a location close to the pulp (nerve) of the tooth. Treatment must be accomplished immediately to save the tooth. Accidents can also cause breakage of the tooth, requiring restoration similar to that required for dental caries.

What is the treatment for dental caries (decay)? At this time, one treatment is accom-

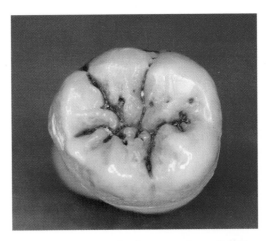

FIG. 18.1 **Grooves on the chewing surfaces of teeth often become decayed; these are usually the first areas to be diseased.**

plished. The diseased part of the tooth is removed with a rotary cutting instrument, air abrader, or laser. You would recognize the rotary instrument as the noisy dental "drill." When you are anesthetized properly, you should not have any discomfort during the dental caries removal stage. The soft, degenerate portion of the tooth is removed by the dentist, leaving only solid, nondecayed tooth structure and a precisely cut tooth preparation that has been designed to retain the restoration (filling) and give proper support to the tooth. The larger and deeper the decayed area, the more difficult it is to treat the tooth successfully and to retain it in the mouth, and the shorter is the time that the restoration can be expected to serve you. At least once every 6 months, routine professional checkups are important for the healthy retention of your teeth.

Tooth restorations will serve for many years if the dental caries has been treated when it is small and the restoration is similarly small. Longevity estimates are made for each type of restoration later in this chapter.

WHAT YOU SEE OR FEEL

Conditions, Signs, or Symptoms Related to Restorative or Operative Dentistry

1. Tooth Is Sensitive to Sweets

Anything that contains sugar, including fruit sugars, causes a sharp, continuing pain from a specific tooth site. This pain usually diminishes over time, or if you rinse well with warm (body temperature) water. Pain caused by sweet foods usually indicates that dental caries (decay) has progressed to a point that it is near the dental pulp (nerve) of the tooth, and you need to seek professional care immediately to reduce the chances of more serious tooth damage, which might require root canal therapy. Depending on the size and depth of the dental caries (decay) in your tooth, one of the described types of restorations (fillings) will usually solve the problem (p. 170).

2. Tooth Is Sensitive to Cold

Ice cream, cold drinks, and other cold foods or drinks cause pain from a specific tooth location. Warming the tooth up reduces the pain. Deep dental caries (decay) often causes sensitivity to cold. Depending on the size and depth of the dental caries in your tooth, one of the described types of restorations (fillings) will usually solve the problem (p. 170).

3. Tooth Is Sensitive to Heat

Hot foods or drinks cause pain for a substantial period or until the tooth reaches body temperature again. This symptom is usually not related to dental caries (decay) but is related most often to a dead or dying dental pulp (nerve) that may require endodontics (root canal therapy) (p. 40).

4. Tooth Is Sensitive to Pressure

Sensitivity to pressure usually indicates a dead or dying dental pulp (nerve) that requires en-

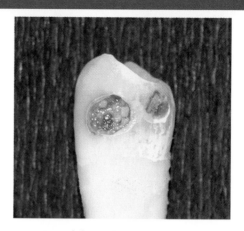

FIG. 18.2 **Typical decayed tooth has external opening caused by dental caries (decay), but internal destruction is much greater in size.**

dodontics (root canal therapy) (p. 40). However, occasionally, impacted food and/or a sweet object in a decayed tooth can cause pain on pressure. Your dentist can tell for sure.

5. Hole in Tooth

Dental caries (decay) starts slowly on the outside surface of a tooth **(FIG. 18.2)**. Often, only a small external hole develops, while the internal portion of the tooth is hollow. The weakened external enamel shell then breaks away, exposing debris and discoloration in the underlying tooth structure. Such a decayed tooth usually requires immediate professional attention to reduce the chance of the need for endodontics (root canal therapy). Depending on the size and depth of the dental caries in your tooth, one of the described types of restorations (fillings) will usually solve the problem (p. 170).

6. Tooth Restoration (Filling) Has Fallen Out

(FIG. 18.3). Most dentists place restorations that have good retention to the tooth structure, and it is unlikely that a restoration will fall out by itself. Sometimes, new decay begins around the edges of a restoration, undermining it and reducing its retention in the remaining tooth structure. As a result, the restoration becomes loose and may eventually fall out. A restoration that comes out usually indicates that the tooth has a significant amount of dental caries (decay) and requires immediate professional care. However, sticky

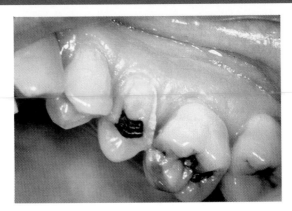

FIG. 18.3   **A piece of the tooth shown has broken off. Patient cannot determine whether a decayed portion has broken off or a filling undermined by decay has come out.**

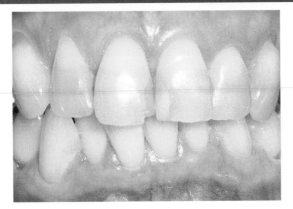

FIG. 18.4   **Upper front teeth have broken and decayed areas that require restorations (fillings). They can be beautifully restored with simple, relatively inexpensive procedures.**

foods such as caramels can pull a restoration out of a tooth. Depending on the size and depth of the decay in your tooth, one of the described types of restorations (fillings) will usually solve the problem (p. 170).

7. Restoration (Filling) Is Loose But Has Not Come Out

Occasionally, restorations (fillings) break, or the tooth structure around them decays further, and a restoration becomes loose in the tooth. This is an especially dangerous condition because the tooth structure cannot be cleaned well. Stagnant food debris and oral plaque collect below the loose restoration, and new decay progresses rapidly. Immediate professional care is mandatory, or the tooth will require endodontics (root canal therapy). Depending on the size and depth of the dental caries (decay), one of the described types of restoration will usually solve the problem (p. 170).

8. Bad Taste Comes From a Tooth When Sucking on It

Dental caries (decay) in an unfilled tooth, or under an existing restoration (filling), collects food debris and degenerating tooth structure, and the result is a foul taste and odor. Dental caries this deep requires immediate professional care. Depending on the size and depth of the dental caries in your tooth, one of the described types of restorations will usually solve the problem (p. 170).

9. Tooth That Was Normal Color Now Has Dark Spot(s)

(FIG. 18.4). Dental caries (decay) undermines the external tooth enamel surface, leaving a hollow cavity underneath. Food debris, food pigments, and tooth degeneration products cause color inside the tooth that usually shows through the external surface. Colors are usually gray, brown, and black. Immediate professional care is needed. Depending on the size and depth of the dental caries in your tooth, one of the described types of restorations (fillings) will usually solve the problem (p. 170).

10. Dental Floss Has a Foul Odor When Removed From Between Teeth

A foul odor on used dental floss can be misinterpreted. Periodontal disease (p. 129), dental caries (decay), or impacted food debris can cause this situation. If one of the other conditions described in this section is present, dental caries (decay) is probably the problem. If none of the other conditions is present, periodontal (gum and bone) disease may be present. If dental caries is present, depending on its size and depth, one of the described types of restorations (fillings) will usually solve the problem (p. 170). If food is impacted, there may be a space between the teeth, requiring a restoration (filling) to help make a tight contact.

11. Notches or Slots at the Gum Line

Notches or slots at the gum line indicate worn, degenerated, or decayed tooth structure. If they are small and shallow, they should probably not be treated unless they are objectionable in appearance. If the notches or slots are decayed or large, they should be restored (filled) immediately to avoid additional damage. Occasionally, incorrect tooth brushing can cause this condition, but more frequently, microscopic bending movements of the tooth caused during chewing cause the notches at the gum line. Depending on the size and depth of the slots or dental caries (decay), one of the described types of restorations (fillings) will usually solve the problem (p. 170).

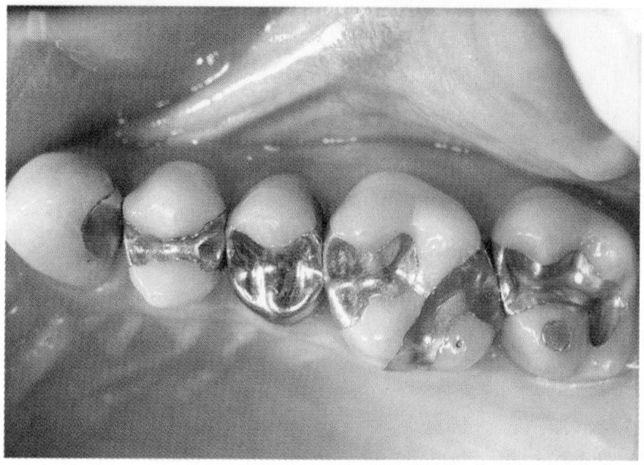

FIG. 18.5   **Several silver restorations are shown. They have been in service 10 to 20 years.**

WHAT YOUR DENTIST CAN DO
Treatment Available

Restoration of teeth (filling teeth) is one of the oldest aspects of dentistry, dating back many hundreds of years. Some of the techniques and materials have been used for a long time, and their service characteristics are well known. Other tooth restorations are much newer, and research is now under way on their serviceability.

Restorations for teeth can be broken down broadly into metallic and tooth-colored restorations. When teeth that are visible during smiling (incisors and canines) need to be restored, tooth-colored materials are usually used, but when teeth in the back of the mouth (premolars and molars) need to be restored, either metallic or tooth-colored materials can be used. The choice is the decision of the patient in consultation with the dentist.

There is now considerable interest in tooth-colored restorations because many people prefer to eliminate metal from their mouths for one or both of the following reasons: (1) better appearance or (2) alleged, but still relatively unproven, negative health characteristics of metals in the body.

Most dental restorations have been silver amalgam, a material that has been used for more than 150 years. However, it is poor in appearance and has other negative characteristics, which are discussed later in this chapter. Tooth-colored composite resin (plastic) is now the most commonly used restoration for front teeth, and its use in back teeth is growing rapidly. The following descriptions will allow you to compare the various types of restorations for teeth.

1. Silver Amalgam
(FIG. 18.5). The most well known and commonly used of all dental restorative materials for back teeth is silver amalgam. It is not acceptable from an appearance standpoint for front teeth. Although it is unsightly and has been indicted for alleged health hazards because of the mercury it contains, silver amalgam continues to be used by the majority of dentists. Most health organizations worldwide accept amalgam as a safe tooth restoration. This material contains silver, tin, copper, and zinc, which are mixed with mercury to form a plastic, compactable mass. When placed into a tooth preparation (refined hole), the material sets to a firm consistency within a few minutes, allowing dentists to shape and carve it. Final strength requires about 24 hours.

   A. **Advantages:** Silver amalgam is the lowest in cost and the longest used of all restorative materials. It is known to serve well for many years in small to moderate size tooth preparations (cavities). It is strong; in fact, it is stronger than natural teeth. Most dentists can place it easily and rapidly.

   B. **Disadvantages:** Silver amalgam ranges in color from shiny silver to gray to black **(FIG. 18.6)**; none of these colors matches tooth color at all. Additionally, over a period of years the silver amalgam imparts a gray color to the surrounding tooth structure, making those teeth that contain silver amalgam look different in overall color from natural teeth. When the silver amalgam is removed from teeth that have turned gray, the natural tooth color returns almost immediately **(FIG. 18.7)**. Silver amalgam cannot be used for teeth that need to match tooth color, or for those that have been destroyed significantly by dental caries or breakage.

C. **Risks:** Although highly controversial, dental silver amalgam has been criticized by some individuals and groups as being toxic because of its mercury content. A growing percentage of dentists in North America will not use this material. All national and international dental societies have affirmed that silver amalgam is safe and should continue to be used, but vociferous groups of anti-amalgam people condemn it.

Many teeth that have had silver amalgam restorations crack over a period of years. In some teeth a portion of the tooth breaks off; others break internally, requiring more comprehensive therapy. Treatment of a cracked tooth varies from a simple restoration (filling) or a crown (cap), to a root canal and crown (cap), to extraction. To help prevent future cracked teeth, many dentists are using new materials to bond the silver to the tooth structure. If a tooth is broken down significantly and your dentist suggests a stronger restoration than silver amalgam (such as a crown [cap]), that suggestion should be accepted.

D. **Alternatives:** Most dentists now use plastic (p. 173) as the most common alternative to silver amalgam. Other alternatives include cast gold inlays and onlays (p. 172), tooth-colored inlays and onlays (p. 174), or crowns (caps) (p. 146).

E. **Cost:** Silver amalgam costs less than all other filling materials, but low cost should not influence you toward this

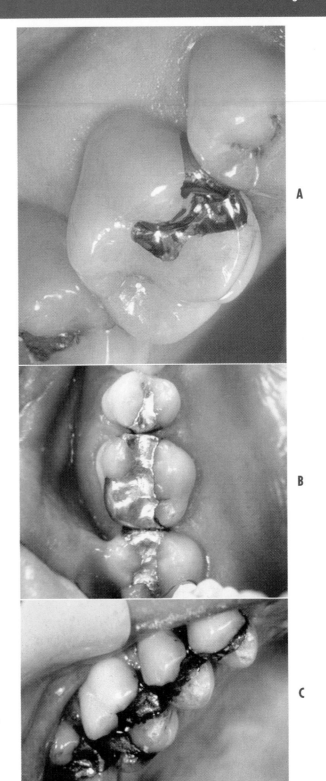

FIG. 18.6   **A,** Smooth, brightly polished silver filling. **B,** Gray, dull but serviceable silver fillings. **C,** Black, tarnished silver fillings, with significant tooth discoloration.

Tooth Restoration

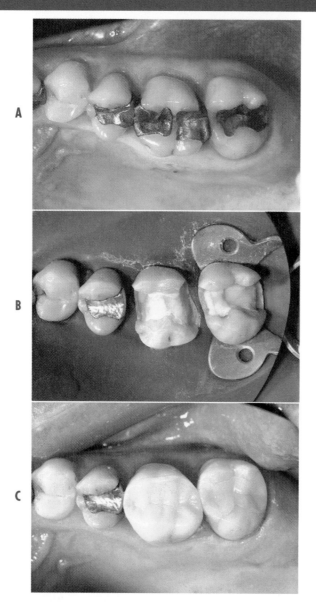

FIG. 18.7   **A,** Old silver fillings. **B,** Silver fillings removed and teeth prepared for tooth-colored restorations. **C,** New restorations made of resin (plastic) are beautiful, and gray color has disappeared from teeth.

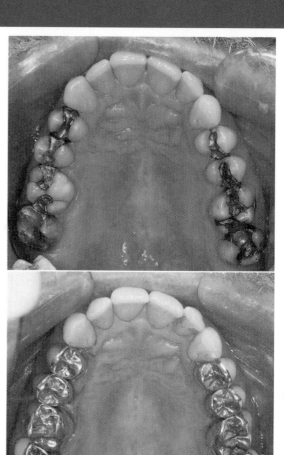

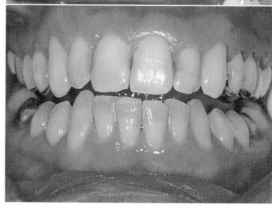

FIG. 18.8   **A,** Patient's upper teeth with previously placed silver amalgam fillings (restorations). **B,** Patient's mouth has been restored with cast gold restoration. **C,** Notice that gold does not show to a significant degree. These restorations should serve most of the patient's life.

restoration if other techniques are suggested because they may be better for your specific situation.

F. **Result of Nontreatment:** Untreated dental caries (decay) will eventually destroy much of the tooth, kill the dental pulp (nerve), and require significant expensive therapy to overcome the problem.

2. Cast Gold Inlays and Onlays

(FIG. 18.8). For nearly a century, cast gold inlays and onlays have been regarded by many dentists as the best, longest-lasting method to repair teeth. Inlays fit within the biting surface of the tooth, whereas onlays cover the top of the biting surface. Many of these restorations serve for most of a patient's lifetime. However, they are difficult to accomplish, expensive, and highly demanding of the dentist's skill.

A. **Advantages:** These restorations may be designed to add strength to weakened teeth by covering weakened portions of teeth. Gold alloys used in dentistry may be designed to wear nearly exactly the way opposing natural tooth enamel wears. This advantage is significant, because opposing teeth are not worn away rapidly. High-quality cast gold restorations have a long service potential.

B. **Disadvantages:** Because of the necessity to make the gold inlay or onlay outside of the mouth in a laboratory, two appointments are necessary. The tooth must first be prepared (trimmed) to remove the decay or old restoration, to allow the inlay or onlay to be placed into or onto the tooth; at a second appointment the restoration is cemented into place. These restorations require significant shaping and cutting of the tooth. Therefore, gold alloy restorations are not as conservative as silver amalgam restorations. Gold alloys are gold in color and are not acceptable to most people in areas of the mouth where they are visible. Their use is generally limited to back teeth.

C. **Risks:** There are no known risks to these restorations, with the possible exception that a very few people may have slight reactions to the metals in gold alloy (e.g., gold, silver, copper, zinc, palladium, platinum).

D. **Alternatives:** In smaller restorations, silver amalgam (p. 170) or composite resin (plastic) (p. 173) are alternatives. For larger restorations, cast gold has no known equivalent except in some form of crown (cap). If a tooth-colored restoration is preferred, tooth-colored inlays and onlays provide a beautiful but less proven alternative.

E. **Cost:** These restorations are expensive because of the dentist's time and effort involved, and the cost of the gold alloy. They are five to eight times more expensive than silver amalgam restorations.

F. **Result of Nontreatment:** Untreated dental caries (decay) will eventually destroy much of the tooth, kill the dental pulp (nerve), and require significant expensive therapy to overcome the problem.

3. Composite Resin (Plastic)

(FIG. 18.9). From a cost standpoint, this tooth-colored restoration is closest to silver amalgam, but composite resin restorations must be placed nearly perfectly to provide adequate service. They can compete with silver amalgam in small to moderate size tooth defects. Many new materials now make these restorations much better than in the past. These are the most common restorations for front teeth.

A. **Advantages:** These restorations are tooth-colored and nonmetallic. When placed over etched enamel, they will bond the remaining tooth structure back together.

B. **Disadvantages:** These restorations must be placed perfectly for optimal service. All materials in this category wear more under biting loads than do metal restorations. However, when appearance is a primary factor, they should be used.

C. **Risks:** A small percentage of teeth into which this material has been placed is sensitive to temperature or pressure after the placement. This sensitivity usually goes away, but a few teeth require endodontic (root canal) therapy because of continued sensitivity. Composite resin wears faster than metals; this characteristic can cause the need for replacement sooner than metals.

D. **Alternatives:** Where appearance is not a factor, silver amalgam is the most used alternative (p. 170), but gold inlays and onlays (p. 172), tooth-colored inlays and onlays (p. 174), and crowns (caps) (p. 146) may also be considered.

E. **Cost:** These restorations may cost up to two or three times more than the cost of silver amalgam restorations in back

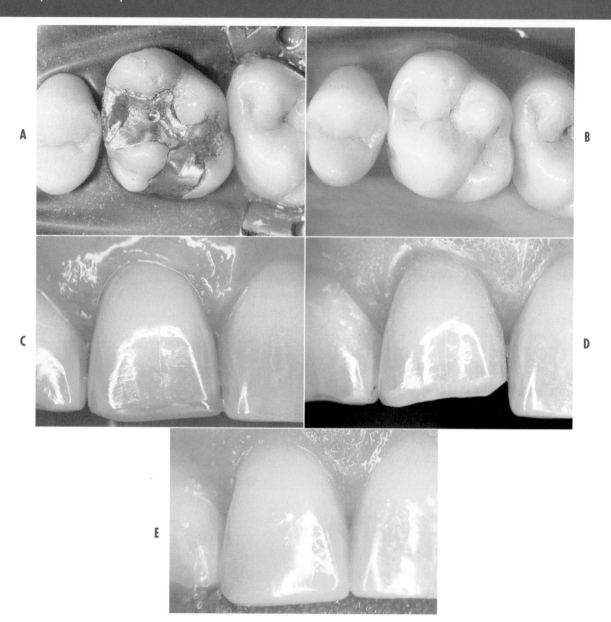

FIG. 18.9   **A,** Silver filling (restoration) in tooth. **B,** Same tooth restored with tooth-colored restoration has been in service 10 years. **C,** Upper front tooth with old discolored filling (restoration). **D,** Old restoration has been removed. **E,** New plastic (resin) restoration has been placed in the tooth. It will serve many years.

teeth, but they are relatively inexpensive for front teeth. The higher cost is related to the extra skill required to place these restorations.

F. **Result of Nontreatment:** Untreated decay will eventually destroy much of the tooth, kill the dental pulp (nerve), and may require significant expensive therapy to overcome the problem.

4. Tooth-Colored Inlays and Onlays

(FIG. 18.10). Several types of tooth-colored inlays and onlays have been developed primar-ily for use in larger defects in back teeth. These are used in place of a crown (cap) or filling (restoration). They are made of porcelain, other ceramics, or resin (plastic). These materials are made in a laboratory and are cemented into place using a liquid plastic form of cement. Two appointments are required for their completion. These are beautiful restorations, matching tooth structure nearly exactly, but they have not been used long enough for optimal research knowledge about their long-term characteristics.

A. **Advantages:** Tooth-colored inlays and

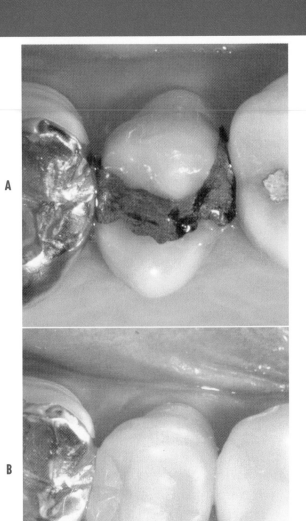

A

B

FIG. 18.10 **A,** Black silver filling to be replaced. **B,** New restoration replacing silver filling is beautiful and functional.

onlays are highly pleasing in appearance and may bond teeth together. They require less removal of tooth structure than a crown (cap).

B. **Disadvantages:** These restorations are not as strong as metallic restorations, and occasional breakage may be expected. They have been used in dentistry for comparatively few years, and knowledge about their long-term service characteristics is lacking.

C. **Risks:** Tooth sensitivity, short or long term, may be present in a few of these restorations. If tooth sensitivity per-

sists, endodontics (root canal therapy) may be necessary, but this is infrequent. Some tooth-colored restorations break during service because they are not as strong as those made of metal. If breakage occurs, the restoration can be remade. Because these restorations have not been used as long as metallic restorations for back teeth, knowledge about long-term service is not complete.

D. **Alternatives:** For back teeth, metallic restorations are the major alternatives. Silver amalgam and cast gold restorations are strong, acceptable alternatives but are not as pleasing in appearance.

E. **Cost:** Usually, these restorations require two appointments and some relatively complex laboratory work. The necessary expertise and effort requires a cost that is near or equal to that of cast gold restorations, or about five to eight times more than silver amalgam restorations.

F. **Result of Nontreatment:** Untreated dental caries (decay) will eventually destroy much of the tooth, kill the dental pulp (nerve), and may require expensive therapy to overcome the problem.

SUMMARY

Restorative or operative dentistry is a major portion of dentistry, because dental caries (decay) has been the most common oral disease. However, most people are not aware of the numerous alternatives for restoring (filling) teeth. Some of these alternatives—composite resin and tooth-colored inlays and onlays—match tooth color well, and clinicians are optimistic about their service potential. Metallic restorations—silver amalgam and cast gold—have been well proven from many years of use and provide known longevity and service. When a significant portion of a tooth has been destroyed, typical restorations (fillings) may not be possible, and crowns (caps) may be necessary. Almost all general dentists and many prosthodontists perform restorative or operative dentistry.

CHAPTER 19

Preventing the Need for Dental Treatment
Protecting Against Future Problems

When you have finished this chapter, you will understand that the need for most dental treatment can be prevented. This is the most valuable chapter in the book, because it describes what you can do to prevent dental disease or injury and thus save yourself future problems, expense, and destruction of your teeth and their supporting structures.

You may know about the standard ways to prevent dental disease and injury, but numerous aspects of this chapter will be new, interesting, and useful to most people. The chapter is organized into subheadings that discuss common preventable situations that cause oral dental disease or injury.

1. **Necessary Oral Hygiene Measures:** Nearly all people think that their oral hygiene is adequate, but most could have much better oral cleaning habits. Cleaning the mouth well helps prevent two major oral diseases: dental caries (decay) and periodontal disease (degeneration of oral bone and gums).

   Tooth brushing accomplishes some oral hygiene requirements. Proper brushing can remove some food debris and dental plaque (sticky, slimy, cream-colored debris that accumulates on tooth surfaces). However, brushing only removes debris from the front, back, and top of the teeth. It does not remove plaque from between the teeth, where a significant amount of dental caries (decay) begins. You must practice oral hygiene between the teeth also, and that requires dental floss. Oral hygiene techniques for a typi-

cal child or adult patient with no major special problems are as follows.

A. **Tooth brushing:** Brushing the teeth after every meal is not excessive, but before bedtime is the most important tooth brushing session. Brushing removes much of the food debris and provides a clean feeling. Unless you have some special allergy or sensitivity problem, fluoride-containing, tartar control toothpaste should be used (FIG. 19.1). You need only a very small amount of toothpaste for each brushing, just enough to flavor the procedure. Be consistent when brushing. Start in a specific place and move systematically around both the front and back sides of the teeth. Avoid back-and-forth horizontal strokes and emphasize up-and-down and circular movements on teeth (FIG. 19.2). Toothbrushes are made in every

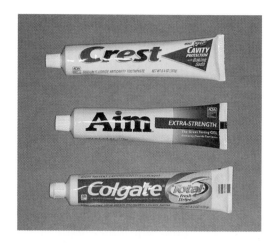

FIG. 19.1   Fluoride-containing, tartar-control tooth-pastes should be used by most people.

shape, size, and color you can imagine (**FIG. 19.3**). However, a soft nylon bristle brush of average size is usually the most satisfactory. Don't use it until it is destroyed—*a few weeks* is enough. Make sure to replace it after a serious illness or an encounter with canker sores. If you do not discard it, you may reinfect yourself. Brushing is only the first step to totally cleaning your mouth.

B. **Dental Flossing:** Flossing is not practiced by enough people. If everybody flossed daily, a significant amount of need for dental therapy could be eliminated because the debris between the teeth, where it cannot be disturbed with a brush, would be eliminated. As with toothbrushes, several types of dental floss are available. Most people find that standard waxed floss is the most acceptable (**FIG. 19.4**); the unwaxed variety catches and frays be-

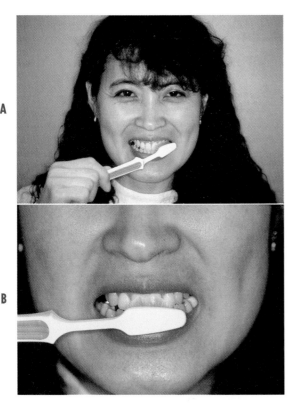

A

B

FIG. 19.2   **A and B,** When brushing, gently roll the toothbrush from the gums to the chewing surface of the teeth in the direction the teeth grow (gums to tooth).

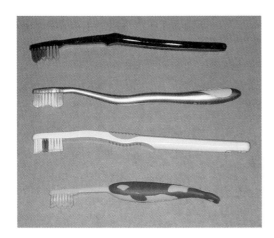

FIG. 19.3   Current popular toothbrushes are excellent. They should be replaced as soon as they appear to be slightly worn or after illness, so you do not reinfect yourself.

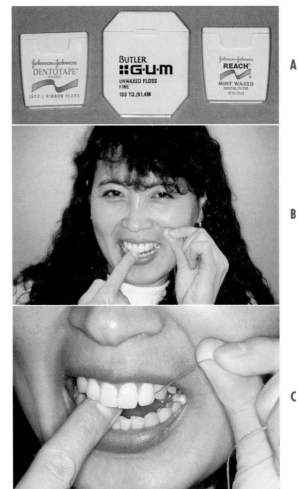

A

B

C

FIG. 19.4   **A to C,** Standard waxed dental floss is best for most people. Flossing at least once every 24 hours, just before bedtime is recommended. Gentle flossing should not injure the gums or produce pain or bleeding.

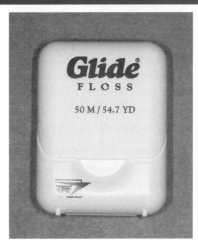

FIG. 19.5 Special, slick, nonshredding floss is available if you tend to fragment floss between your teeth.

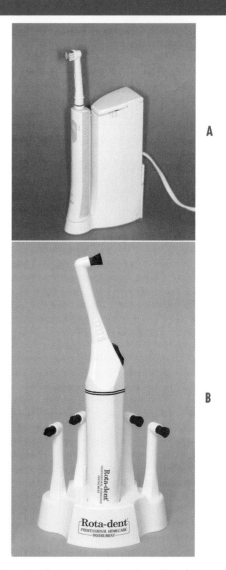

FIG. 19.6 **A,** The Braun mechanical toothbrush is one of the most popular on the market. Mechanical toothbrushes are a major help to patients who have difficulty using their hands. **B,** The Rota-dent was one of the first mechanical toothbrushes to provide a rotating brush that easily reaches areas difficult to access. It has been well accepted.

tween the teeth of many people. If the floss catches between your teeth, see your dentist for smoothing. Also, new types of floss that do not shred are now available **(FIG. 19.5).** Floss should be used at least once daily, and the best time is just before bedtime. Debris accumulated on the teeth that stays undisturbed during sleeping can be hazardous to your teeth if allowed to continue. Many people do not use floss correctly. The floss should be placed gently between the tooth contact areas and then slipped between the gums and the tooth on both sides of the gum (papilla) between each tooth.

C. **Mechanical Toothbrushes:** Some people need mechanical toothbrushes. If you do not like to brush your teeth and find that you neglect the task often, or that you are not thorough in carrying it out, a mechanical toothbrush may be best for you. If you are physically disabled with your hands, or if you know someone who has a mental disability that does not allow them to understand the need for oral care, a mechanical toothbrush is necessary. If you have a friend or relative with natural teeth who is ill or debilitated and living in a nursing home, a mechanical toothbrush could be helpful. Almost any mechanical toothbrush can be better than a manual toothbrush for most people, but at least two brands have achieved significant acceptance. Braun and Rota-dent toothbrushes **(FIG. 19.6)** are examples of mechanical toothbrushes that can provide optimal cleaning capability when used properly.

D. **Special Cleaners:** Certain cleaners that allow access to difficult areas of the mouth and between teeth **(FIGS. 19.7 and 19.8)** are needed by some persons with special oral cleaning needs. Ask your

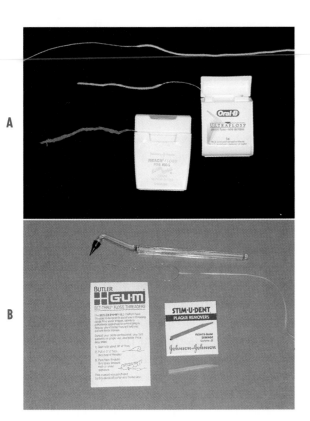

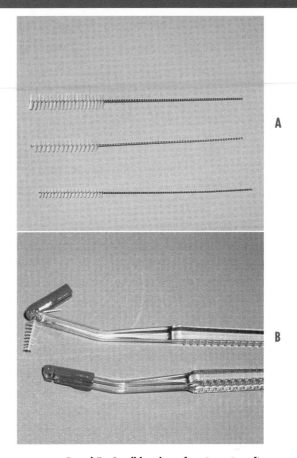

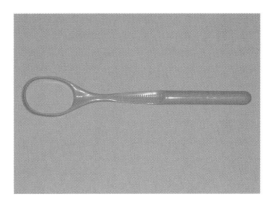

FIG. 19.7   A, These special cleaning products assist patients who have spaces between their teeth or have bridges in place. **B,** Small toothpick and bridge threaders help patients clean in difficult situations.

FIG. 19.8   A and B, Small brushes of various sizes fit well in situations in which there is significant space between teeth. Consult with your dentist; you may need them.

dentist or dental hygienist about your particular needs.

E. **Tongue Cleaning: (FIG. 19.9).** In many people, the tongue is covered with food debris and microorganisms. About 50% of the population needs to clean their tongues daily. Research has shown that the taste buds on some tongues are long enough to collect debris and microorganisms and cause bad breath. It has been estimated that the majority of bad breath is caused by tongue debris. Tooth brushing does not remove this debris, and brushing the tongue does not remove the debris well either. Pull your tongue out. If it is gray and has obvious debris on it, you need a tongue scraper.

Tongue scrapers are readily available in the oral hygiene departments of stores.

FIG. 19.9   Tongue cleaners remove many of the organisms that cause decay, gum disease, and bad breath.

They are easy to use. You place the device as far back in your mouth as comfort allows, press firmly, and pull the scraper forward. After using the scraper, your mouth will feel clean, your breath will be

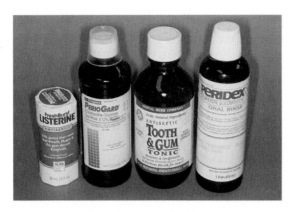

FIG. 19.10 *Many antimicrobiological mouth rinses reduce microorganisms and bad breath.*

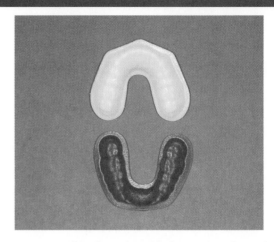

FIG. 19.11 *Fluoride can be applied in trays to the teeth. This preventive treatment should be accomplished for children once every 6 months.*

fresher, and tooth decay and gum disease should be reduced.

F. **Mouthwashes:** (FIG. 19.10) Many mouthwashes currently are on the market. Most of these solutions taste good, and they make your mouth feel clean. Research has shown that their positive influence on breath odor varies from a few minutes to less than 1 hour.

Some nonprescription mouthwashes have a minor therapeutic influence on either dental decay or periodontal disease. Weak fluoride rinses can be obtained without a prescription and provide a small positive preventive therapy.

Your dentist can prescribe very strong fluoride or antimicrobiological mouthwashes for dental decay or periodontal disease. These strong rinses are helpful in controlling oral disease.

2. **Fluoride:** One of the most proven public health measures in the history of medicine is the use of fluoride to help prevent dental caries (decay). In fact, dental decay has been remarkably reduced around the world over the past 50 years because of the placement of small amounts of fluoride into various agents that enter the body, as described later. Nearly all persons with natural teeth should use toothpaste-containing fluoride. Be suspicious

of the motives of various individuals or groups that have attempted to eliminate the use of fluoride for prevention of dental caries. How much fluoride and in what form is it needed in addition to fluoride toothpaste?

A. **Children** need fluoride either supplied in their drinking water or as a supplement to their diet. Check with your dentist or dental hygienist to see if the water you drink contains an acceptable amount of fluoride. If it does not, check to find the best method to supplement the diet. Children who receive optimal levels of fluoride from birth to early teens have minimal, if any, dental caries (decay). Fluoride supplements for children can be in vitamins, separate tablets, or as a liquid delivered in water or juice. However, fluoride needs to be carefully controlled to avoid overdosage because of the routine use of fluoride in toothpastes and rinses. Check with your dentist concerning optimal amounts of fluoride for your child. Children who live in nonfluoridated areas should have fluoride applied topically to their teeth using trays (FIG. 19.11) at least once every 6 months.

B. **Teenagers** are often negligent in carrying out oral hygiene. Therefore, making certain that optimal fluoride is present in

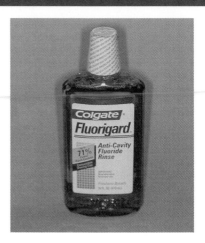

FIG. 19.12   Fluoride rinses reduce dental caries (decay) and should be used by almost all persons except small children.

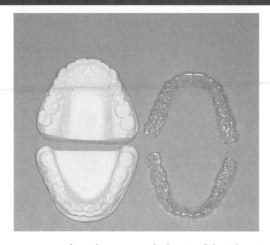

FIG. 19.13   If you have a very high rate of dental caries (decay), your dentist may prescribe individually fitted trays that provide high levels of fluoride to your teeth once per day. This procedure can stop new caries (decay).

their mouths can help prevent dental caries despite their poor oral hygiene. After the permanent teeth have developed, there appears to be no need for fluoride in the diet, which has already been deposited into the teeth as they formed. However, there is a significant need for a fluoride solution to come in contact with the teeth daily in the form of oral rinses. This fluoride reduces the chance of tooth decay by strengthening the surface layers of the teeth. Many fluoride rinses are available for purchase by the general public in grocery stores or pharmacies. Some popular brand names are Fluorigard (Colgate) or ACT (Johnson and Johnson) (FIG. 19.12). These solutions used daily as a rinse (preferably just before bedtime) reduce dental caries on smooth surfaces of teeth by about 40%. Such solutions used as rinses are suggested for everybody with natural teeth. Occasionally, stronger rinses or brush-on fluoride is needed, or even fluoride applied to the teeth in specially fitted plastic trays (FIG. 19.13) that hold the fluoride in close contact to the teeth for a specified time. If dental caries is a major problem in a teenager, your dentist or hygienist should suggest and supervise the use of strong fluoride applications (FIG. 19.14).

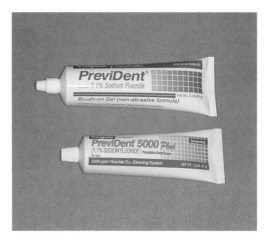

FIG. 19.14   Strong fluoride is necessary for people with a high rate of dental caries (decay). See your dentist if this is your problem.

C. **Adults** need fluoride applied to the surfaces of their teeth as rinses. The standard rinses described above for teenagers are suggested as routine daily applications for adults also. Older adults, or those with diseases that have degenerated their overall health significantly, need strong fluoride rinses, brushed-on fluoride, or fluoride in special form-fitted trays used daily (described above for teenagers).

D. **Mature adults** need more fluoride than young and middle-aged adults, because their tooth-supporting structures (bone

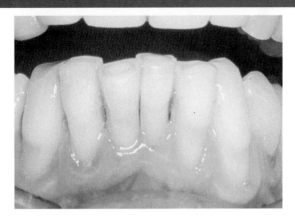

FIG. 19.15 Gums have receded on the lower teeth, exposing the tooth root surfaces.

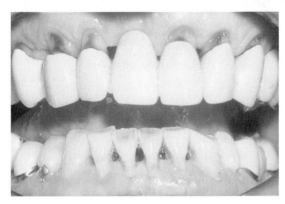

FIG. 19.17 Severe dental decay where gums have receded, exposing tooth root surfaces.

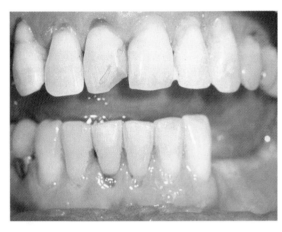

FIG. 19.16 Dental decay has started on the tooth root surfaces where the gums have receded. This is especially difficult to control; see your dentist if this occurs.

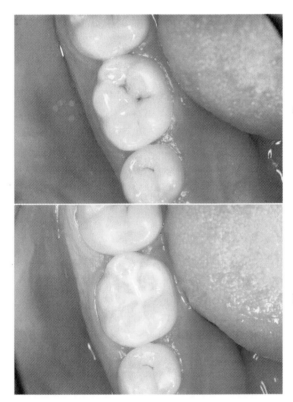

FIG. 19.18 **A,** Black pits and fissures on chewing surfaces of teeth. **B,** Pits and fissures have been sealed on center tooth, preventing decay in that area. Most children need at least some sealants.

and gums) have receded, leaving root surfaces of the teeth exposed to oral debris (**FIGS. 19.15** and **19.16**). These root surfaces become decayed extremely rapidly and easily, thus causing a painful and difficult-to-treat condition common in mature adults: root caries (**FIG. 19.17**). Fluoride rinses, brush-on fluoride, or fluoride in trays is indicated for many mature adults.

3. **Sealants:** All teeth develop by having enamel grow and accumulate on their surfaces from the inside of the tooth to the outside. When the enamel portions do not connect completely during tooth development, pits or fissures form (**FIG. 19.18, A**), especially on the chewing surfaces of the back teeth (molars and pre-

molars). These teeth should be sealed with small amounts of plastic at appropriate times (**FIG. 19.18, B**) beginning at about age 6. When the sealant procedure is accomplished, dental caries on the chewing surfaces of the teeth is greatly reduced or eliminated.

4. **Regular Professional Checkups and Care:** Most persons should consult with a dentist at least once every 6 months. Many disease situations arise so rapidly that even 6 months is too long, and some patients require checkups once every 4 months. The visit should include a cleaning of your teeth, a thorough visual examination, dental radiographs (x-rays) when needed, and an examination of your jawbone, gums, jaw joints, and oral soft tissues. Although public hysteria about x-rays has occurred, there is no reason to avoid dental x-rays when needed. Some persons require radiographs once every 6 months, others less frequently. You receive more x-ray dosage in a short time standing in the sun or riding in an airplane than you get from most dental x-rays. Asking your dentist to diagnose a problem in your mouth without x-rays is similar to asking your automobile mechanic to diagnose the problem with a faulty engine without raising the car hood. Patients who neglect routine oral checkups should expect more expensive and less repairable oral problems when they are eventually forced to visit a dentist for treatment.

5. **Diet:** Diet is highly important relative to oral diseases. A good, balanced diet improves the possibility that oral structures will develop well and maintain themselves throughout life. Several simple factors can reduce your chances of having dental caries or periodontal disease (gum and bone degeneration):

A. Avoid excessive amounts of sugar-containing foods **(FIG. 19.19)**.

B. When eating sugar-containing foods, do so during meals, and clean your mouth thoroughly immediately afterward.

C. Avoid constant snacks. Limit eating to two or three meals per day, and clean your mouth after each. Frequent eating of sugar-containing foods without brushing will result in dental disease.

D. Avoid constant sipping of high-sugar beverages such as soft drinks, fruit juice, or sweetened coffee.

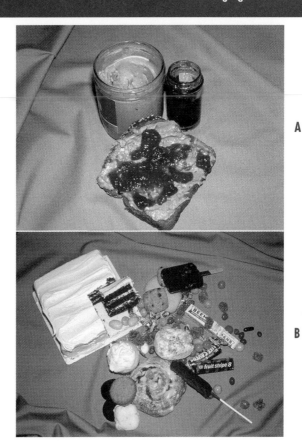

FIG. 19.19   A and B, The diet of many people contains amazingly high levels of sugar. Not only is sugar terrible for teeth, but also it is not a good food source and causes several other systemic disease conditions. Reduce it!

E. Avoid sticky foods such as caramels, dates, and graham crackers. Food that sticks to teeth causes more dental disease than similar amounts of sugar in less sticky forms or in liquids.

Normal, healthy foods **(FIG. 19.20)** eaten two or three times per day and cleaned from teeth after eating do not stimulate dental disease.

6. **Grinding Teeth:** If you have the habit of bruxism or clenching **(FIG. 19.21)** (p. 76), and you grind your teeth when you are not eating, you can expect up to 80 times the normal tooth wear per day compared with normal nonbruxing/clenching persons. About one fourth to one third of the overall population has this unfortunate condition. If the condition is diagnosed early in life, the destruction to the dentition that it inevitably causes without

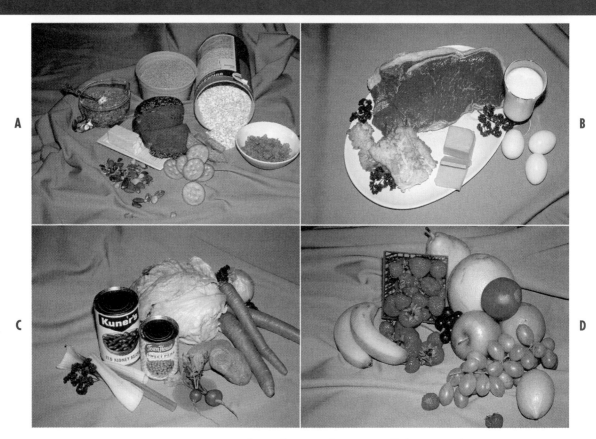

FIG. 19.20 **A** to **D,** Persons who emphasize moderate, controlled amounts of normally accepted foods soon find not only that their oral conditions improved, but also that their overall health is better. Avoid excesses of any foods and large quantities of sugar and fat. Clean your mouth preferably after every meal.

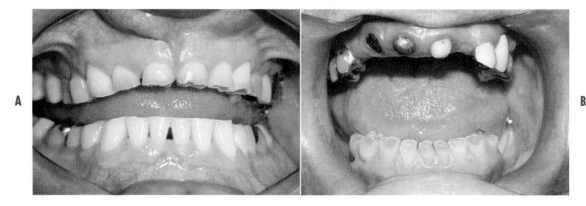

FIG. 19.21 **A,** At least 30% of the population grinds their teeth excessively, producing the result shown after a few years. **B,** This person chewed so aggressively that the upper front teeth were destroyed and the lower teeth were worn severely.

treatment can be slowed or prevented completely by use of night guards or other therapy (FIG. 19.22).

7. **Athletics:** Football, basketball, soccer, racquetball, rugby, water skiing, snow skiing,

softball, baseball, and many other sports provide the constant risk to participants of forceful contact with other persons, balls, the ground, or other obstacles. Occasionally, teeth are fractured, broken off,

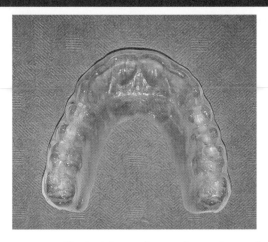

FIG. 19.22 **Plastic night guards control excessive tooth wear. You may need one—ask your dentist.**

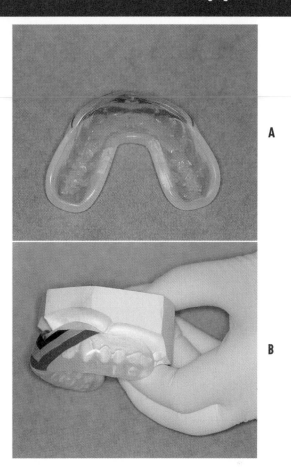

A

B

FIG. 19.24 **A and B,** Wear an athletic mouth guard if you participate in such activities!

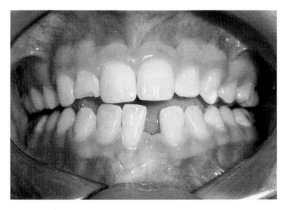

FIG. 19.23 **The lower tooth was knocked out and lost in an athletic event.**

or knocked out during athletic activity **(FIG. 19.23)**. However, a less well-known result of such participation is the development of hundreds of small microscopic cracks in teeth that go relatively unobserved until later in life, when pieces of tooth break off.

Persons involved in active sports should ask their dentist to make an athletic mouth guard to help prevent the development of irreversible damage to tooth structure during these enjoyable but potentially dangerous activities **(FIG. 19.24)**.

8. **Accidents:** All of us try to prevent having an accident that might damage any part of our bodies, but damage to the head is to be especially avoided **(FIG. 19.25)**. When you participate in any high-risk ac-tivity such as bicycle, motorcycle, or horseback riding; driving an automobile; or hundreds of other activities, you should use the necessary protective measures (helmets, seat belts, straps, etc.) to avoid damage to the body. Teeth are strong, but they are brittle. A blow to the body can force the teeth together, cracking, breaking, or dislodging them, and damage to teeth does not heal. When they are damaged, only a dentist can repair or replace them.

9. **Aggressive Chewing of Hard Objects:** Occasionally, we all encounter biting a hard object such as a chicken bone, a piece of stone, sand, or other substance in food, and the shock is startling. The teeth have very sensitive nerves. For this reason, toothaches can be highly painful. Pain from teeth and their supporting structures warns you that you are exceeding

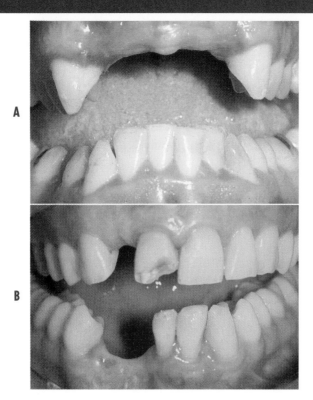

A

B

FIG. 19.25 **A** and **B,** Two accident victims whose tooth repair was time-consuming and expensive. Be careful— your body parts are difficult, if not impossible, to replace.

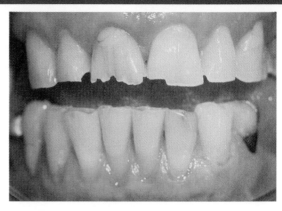

FIG. 19.26 **Breakage of teeth caused by opening hair-pins with the front teeth.**

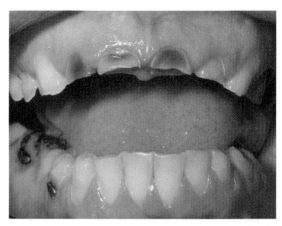

FIG. 19.27 **The destruction of dentition in the mouth of this 26-year-old woman was caused by the eat-and-purge syndrome, bulimia.**

the desirable stress on your teeth. However, some persons purposely chew hard objects such as hard candy, ice, peanut brittle, popcorn, corn nuts, and other items. The damage caused to teeth by chewing these objects is clearly observable. You may certainly eat such objects, but the haste with which you eat them relates directly to the damage you cause to your teeth. It is suggested that you dissolve hard candies in your mouth instead of cracking them with your teeth, that you melt ice in your mouth instead of biting it, and that you soften popcorn or corn nuts in your mouth for a while before gently biting them. The teeth of an ice chewer or a person who practices other aggressive chewing are evident to a dentist immediately by the cracks, broken pieces, worn fillings, and overall aged appearance **(FIG. 19.26).** Don't do it!

10. **Eating Disorders:** An increasingly common malady of modern affluent society is the eat-and-purge disease, bulimia **(FIG. 19.27).** Such abnormal constant regurgitation places acid on teeth surfaces and dissolves the superficial enamel tooth structure in a few months to a few years. When the tooth structure is gone, crowns (caps) and/or other therapy must be used to rebuild the dentition. Most people who have this disease would prefer to stop, and damage to teeth should be another reason to do so. Professional psychological and dental help should be obtained to help control various aspects of the disease.

11. **Smoking:** Smoking is responsible for yet another human misfortune; smokers are more likely to develop periodontal disease. The gums and oral tissues of a smoker are bright red. This chronic

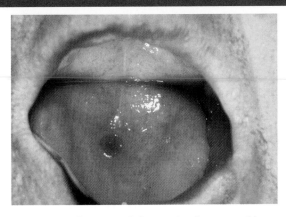

FIG. 19.28   **The cancer of this man's palate, caused by smoking, resulted in the loss of his palate, part of his nose, and one eye. Is there really any reason to smoke? (This is a mirror view.)**

inflammation contributes to constant breakdown of soft tissues and subsequent underlying bone destruction. Additionally, smoking is the leading cause of oral cancer **(FIG. 19.28)**, another reason to break this harmful habit.

12. **Smokeless Tobacco:** Chewing tobacco causes increased dental caries because it contains sugar. Further, it is a leading cause of oral cancer at the site where the wad of tobacco is held during chewing. This habit is growing among young persons. Elimination of the habit slows dental caries and reduces the potential development of oral cancer later.

SUMMARY

The body and all its parts are fragile. When a part of your body is damaged or destroyed, you cannot easily return it to the preaccident status. Prevention is always better than treatment, and preventing most oral disease is possible today. If a child born at this time has periodic professional observation, fluoride application, proper oral hygiene, a good diet, and sealants, and avoids the other conditions presented in this chapter, then his or her dentition and its supporting structures should remain healthy throughout life. The choice is yours.

Preventing Dental Problems

CHAPTER 20

Additional Sources of Information

This book was written in simple language to allow readers to obtain and use the information rapidly and easily. However, some persons may want to further extend their knowledge. The following sources provide in-depth information about every area of dentistry and include reference books, professional dental organizations, dental schools, and professional dental organizations (geographic constituent societies).

Such references are available for every country; however, North America is emphasized in this book.

CURRENT BOOKS

Although written for dental students, graduate students, and dentists, most information in these books is understandable to most interested lay readers as well. Every specialty, area, or division in dentistry is represented. You may find most of these books in dental or medical school libraries, or you may ask your local public librarian where the desired book(s) may be obtained. The books are listed by specific clinical areas:

Anesthesia

1. *Management of Pain and Anxiety in the Dental Office,* 2002. R Dionne, D Becker, J Phero (WB Saunders).

Endodontics

1. *Pathways of the Pulp,* ed 8, 2002. S Cohen and RC Burns (Mosby).

2. *Problem Solving in Endodontics,* ed 3, 1997. JL Gutmann, TC Dumsha, PE Lovdahl, EJ Hovland (Mosby).

3. *Endodontic Surgery,* 1993. CR Stockdale (Quintessence).

4. *Color Atlas of Endodontics,* 2002. WT Johnson (Mosby).

Esthetic Dentistry

1. *Esthetic Composite Bonding,* ed 2, 1993. RE Jordan (Mosby).

2. *Aesthetic Dentistry With Indirect Resins,* 1992. H Stean (Quintessence).

3. *Change Your Smile,* ed 3, 1997. RE Goldstein (Quintessence).

Implant Dentistry

1. *Contemporary Implant Dentistry,* ed 2, 1999. CE Misch (Mosby).

2. *Dental Implants: Are They for Me?* ed 2, 1993. TD Taylor (Quintessence).

3. *The Branemark Osseointegrated Implant,* 1989. T Albrektsson and GA Zarb (Quintessence).

4. *Dental Implants: the Art and Science,* 2001. C Babbush (WB Saunders).

5. *Atlas of Oral Implantology,* ed 2, 1999. AN Cranin, M Klein, AM Simons (Mosby).

Occlusion

1. *Management of Temporomandibular Disorders and Occlusion,* ed 4, 1998. JP Okeson (Mosby).

2. *Evaluation, Diagnosis, and Treatment*

of Occlusal Problems, ed 2, 1989. PE Dawson (Mosby).

3. *Current Controversies in Temporomandibular Disorders,* 1994. C McNeil (Quintessence).

Oral and Maxillofacial Surgery, Oral Pathology, Oral Medicine

1. *A Colour Atlas of Orofacial Diseases,* ed 2, 1991. WR Tyldesley (Mosby).
2. *Colour Atlas of Oral Disease,* ed 2, 1994. RA Cawson et al (Mosby).
3. *Atlas of Minor Oral Surgery,* 2001. H Dym and O Ogle (WB Saunders).
4. *Atlas of Oral and Maxillofacial Pathology,* 2000. JA Regezi, JJ Sciubba, MA Pogrel (WB Saunders).
5. *Differential Diagnosis of Oral Lesions,* ed 5, 1997. NK Wood and PM Goaz (Mosby).
6. *Dentofacial Deformities: Integrated Orthodontics & Surgical Correction,* vol 4, ed 2, 1999. BN Epker, JP Stella, LC Fish (Mosby).

Orthodontics

1. *Contemporary Orthodontics,* ed 3, 2000. WR Proffit and HW Fields, Jr. (Mosby).
2. *Orthodontics: Current Principles and Techniques,* ed 3, 2000. TM Graber and RL Vanarsdall Jr (Mosby).
3. *Current Controversies in Orthodontics,* 1991. B Melsen (Quintessence).

Pediatric Dentistry

1. *Colour Guide Orthodontics and Paediatric Dentistry,* 2000. D Millett and RR Welbury (Churchill Livingstone).
2. *Dentistry for the Child and Adolescent,* ed 7, 1999. RE McDonald and DR Avery (Mosby).

Periodontics

1. *Contemporary Periodontics,* 1990. RJ Genco, HM Goldman, W Cohen (Mosby).
2. *Carranza's Clinical Periodontology,* ed 9, 2002. MG Newman, FA Carranza Jr, and H Takei (WB Saunders).

Prosthodontics, Fixed

1. *Planning and Making Crowns and Bridges,* ed 3, 1998. BGN Smith (Mosby).
2. *Contemporary Fixed Prosthodontics,* ed 3, 2001. SF Rosenstiel et al (Mosby).

Prosthodontics, Removable

1. *An Atlas of Removable Partial Denture Design,* 1988. Stratton and Wiebelt (Quintessence).

Radiography

1. *Dental Radiography: Principles and Techniques,* ed 2, 2000. JI Haring and L Jansen (WB Saunders).

Restorative Dentistry or Operative Dentistry

1. *Essentials of Traumatic Injuries to the Teeth,* ed 2, 2000. JO Andreasen (Mosby).
2. *The Art and Science of Operative Dentistry,* ed 4, 2002. TM Roberson and H Heymann (Mosby).
3. *Successful Restorative Dentistry,* 2001. D Walmsley, P Drummer, T Walsh (Churchill Livingstone).

PROFESSIONAL DENTAL ORGANIZATIONS FOR SPECIFIC SUBJECT AREAS

Every division in dentistry has professional organizations that represent their specific areas. Questions about practitioners in your area (or any other question) may be referred to these sources.

National Dental Organizations

The following addresses are maintained by the Department of Dental Society Services, 211 East Chicago Avenue, Chicago, IL 60611, 312/440-2600. Annual meeting dates for national dental organizations are included in the publication, *Calendar of Dental Meetings,* published by the Council on ADA Sessions and International Relations. A copy can be obtained by contacting the council at 312/440-2658.

For More Information

Academy for Implants & Transplants
Executive Director: Dr. Jonathan Lillard
7015 Old Keene Mill Road
Springfield, VA 22150
703/451-0001

Academy for Sports Dentistry
Executive Director: Mrs. Susan D. Ferry
Otolaryngology Department
University Hospital & Clinics
Iowa City, IA 52242
800/273-1788

Academy of Dental Materials
President: Dr. Robert L. Erikson
6101 Lynn Way
Woodbury, MN 55129
612/733-2071

Academy of Dentistry for Persons with Disabilities
Executive Director: Dr. Michael A. Siegel
211 East Chicago Avenue
Fifth Floor
Chicago, IL 60611
312/440-2660

Academy of Dentistry International
3813 Gordon Creek Drive
PO Box 307
Hicksville, OH 43526
419/542-0101

Academy of General Dentistry
Executive Director: Mr. Harold E. Donnell Jr.,
　CAE
211 East Chicago Avenue
Suite 1200
Chicago, IL 60611
312/440-4300

Academy of Laser Dentistry
Executive Director: Ms. Gail Siminovski
Suite 440
9629 Westview Drive
Coral Springs, FL 33076
954/356-3776

Academy of LDS Dentists
Course Coordinator: Mr. Steve Trost
Brigham Young University
Conferences and Workshops
147 HCEB
Provo, UT 84602
801/378-2536

Academy of Operative Dentistry
President: Dr. Ebb A. Berry III
PO Box 177
Menomonie, WI 54751
602/248-9445

Academy of Oral Dynamics
President: Dr. Bertram Kreger
134 East Church Road
Elkins Park, PA 19027
215/635-2336

Academy of Osseointegration
Executive Director: Mr. Kevin Smith
Suite 550
85 West Algonquin Road
Arlington Heights, IL 60005
800/656-7736

Academy of Prosthodontics
Secretary/Treasurer: Dr. Edward J. Plekavich
4830 V Street NW
Washington, DC 20007
202/342-0442

Alliance of American Dental Association
Executive Director: Ms. Kathy Cooper
211 East Chicago Avenue, Fifth Floor
Chicago, IL 60611
312/440-2865

Alpha Omega International Dental Fraternity
Executive Director: Ms. Stephanie Block
Suite 206
1314 Bedford Avenue
Baltimore, MD 21208-3707
410/602-3300

American Academy of Cosmetic Dentistry
Executive Director: Dr. Kenneth L.
  Zakariasen
Suite 200
2810 Walton Commons West
Madison, WI 53718
608/222-8583

American Academy of Dental Electrosurgery
Executive Director: Dr. Maurice J Oringer
15 West 81st Street
New York, NY 10024
212/595-1925

American Academy of Dental Group Practice
Executive Director: Dr. Robert Hankin
2525 East Arizona Biltmore Circle
Suite 127
Phoenix, AZ 85016
602/381-1185

American Academy of Dental Practice Administration
Executive Director: Ms. Kathleen Uebel
1063 South Whippoorwill Lane
Palatine, IL 60067
847/934-4404

American Academy of Esthetic Dentistry
Executive Director: Mr. Tom Stautzenbach
401 North Michigan Avenue
Suite 2400
Chicago, IL 60611
312/321-5121

American Academy of Fixed Prosthodontics
President: Dr. Robert S. Staffanou
PO Box 1409
Bodega Bay, CA 94923
707/875-3040

American Academy of Gnathologic Orthopedics
Executive Director: Ms. Barbara Lopez
2651 Oak Grove Road
Walnut Creek, CA 94598
925/939-5024

American Academy of Gold Foil Operators
Executive Director: Dr. Ronald K. Harris
17922 Tailgrass Court
Noblesville, IN 46060
317/867-0414

American Academy of Implant Dentistry
Executive Director: Mr. J. Vincent Shuck
211 East Chicago Avenue
750
Chicago, IL 60611
312/335-1550

American Academy of Maxillofacial Prosthetics
Executive Director: Dr. Thomas R. Cowper
Cleveland Clinic Foundation
Department of Dentistry
9500 Euclid Avenue
Cleveland, OH 44195
216/444-2084

American Academy of Oral & Maxillofacial Pathology
Executive Director: Ms. Jeanette L. Helfrich
Suite 600
710 East Ogden Avenue
Naperville, IL 60563
630/369-2406

American Academy of Oral & Maxillofacial Radiology
Executive Secretary: Dr. M. Kevin O. Carroll
University of Mississippi
School of Dentistry
2500 North State Street
Jackson, MS 39216
601/984-6060

American Academy of Oral Medicine
Executive Director: Dr. Abraham Reiner
c/o Ms. Joyce Caplan
2910 Lightfoot Drive
Baltimore, MD 21209
410/602-8585

American Academy of Orofacial Pain
Executive Director: Ms. Dale Zeigler
19 Mantula Road
Mount Royal, NJ 08061
609/423-3629

For More Information

American Academy of Orthodontics for the General Practitioner
Executive Director: Ms. Marlene Cayugan
920 Bascom Hill Drive
Baraboo, WI 53913-1281
800/499-0300

American Academy of Pediatric Dentistry
Executive Director: Dr. John S. Rutkauskas
Suite 700
211 East Chicago Avenue
Chicago, IL 60611
312/337-2169

American Academy of Periodontology
Executive Director: Ms. Alice Deforest, CAE
737 North Michigan Avenue
Suite 800
Chicago, IL 60611
312/787-5518

American Academy of Restorative Dentistry
President: Dr. William H. McHorris
1184 College Avenue
Elko, NV 89801
775/738-7165

American Association for Dental Research
Executive Director: Dr. Eli Schwarz
1619 Duke Street
Alexandria, VA 22314-3406
703/548-0066

American Association of Dental Consultants
Executive Director: Ms. Judy Salisbury
PO Box 3345
Lawrence, KS 66046
913/749-1772

American Association of Dental Editors
Executive Director: Mr. Detlef B. Moore
735 North Water Street
Suite 617
Milwaukee, WI 53202
414/272-2759

American Association of Dental Examiners
Executive Director: Ms. Molly Nadler
211 East Chicago Avenue
Suite 760
Chicago, IL 60611
312/440-7464

American Association of Endodontists
Executive Director: Ms. Irma S. Kudo
211 East Chicago Avenue
Suite 1100
Chicago, IL 60611
312/266-7255

American Association of Hospital Dentists
Executive Director: Dr. John Rutkauskas
211 East Chicago Avenue, Fifth Floor
Chicago, IL 60611
312/440-2660

American Association of Oral & Maxillofacial Surgeons
Executive Director: Dr. Robert C. Rinaldi
9700 West Bryn Mawr Avenue
Rosemont, IL 60018
847/678-6200

American Association of Orthodontists
Executive Director: Mr. Ronald Moen
401 North Lindbergh Boulevard
Saint Louis, MO 63141
314/993-1700

American Association of Public Health Dentistry
Executive Director: Dr. James Toothaker
National Office
3760 SW Lyle Court
Portland, OR 97221
503/242-0712

American Association of Stomatologists
President: Dr. Jed Jacobsen
University of Michigan
School of Dentistry
Department of Oral Diagnosis
Ann Arbor, MI 48109
313/763-3316

American Association of Women Dentists
Executive Director: Ms. Sharon Goutschy
401 North Michigan Avenue
Suite 800
Chicago, IL 60611
312/280-9296

American Board of Dental Public Health
Executive Director: Dr. Stanley Lotzkar
1321 NW 47th Terrace
Gainesville, FL 32605
325/378-6301

American Board of Endodontics
Executive Director: Ms. Margie Hannen
211 East Chicago Avenue
Suite 1150
Chicago, IL 60611
312/266-7310

American Board of Oral & Maxillofacial Pathology
Executive Director: Ms. Clarita Wendrich
4320 North Kennedy Boulevard
Suite 690
Tampa, FL 33622
813/286-2444

American Board of Oral & Maxillofacial Surgery
Executive Director: Ms. Cheryl Mounts
625 North Michigan Avenue
Suite 1820
Chicago, IL 60611
312/642-0070

American Board of Orthodontics
Executive Secretary: Ms. Christine L.
   Eisenmayer
401 North Lindbergh Boulevard, #308
Saint Louis, MO 63141
314/432-6130

American Board of Pediatric Dentistry
Executive Director: Dr. James R. Roche
1193 Woodgate Drive
Carmel, IN 46033
317/573-0877

American Board of Periodontology
Executive Director: Dr. Gerald M. Bowers
4157 Mountain Road
Suite 249
Pasadena, MD 21122
410/437-3749

American Board of Prosthodontics
Executive Director: Dr. William Culpepper
PO Box 8437
Atlanta, GA 31106
404/876-2625

American Cleft Palate-Craniofacial Association
Executive Director: Ms. Nancy Smythe
104 South Estes Drive
Suite 204
Chapel Hill, NC 27514
919/933-9044

American College of Dentists
Executive Director: Dr. Stephen Ralls
839 Quince Orchard Boulevard, #J
Gaithersburg, MD 20878
301/977-3223

American College of Oral & Maxillofacial Surgeons
Executive Director: Ms. Emelie C. Schnettler
1100 NW Loop 410
Suite 506
San Antonio, TX 78213
210/344-5674

American College of Prosthodontics
Executive Director: Mr. Stephen D. Hines
211 East Chicago Avenue
Suite 1000
Chicago, IL 60611
312/573-1260

American Dental Assistants' Association
Executive Director: Mr. Lawrence H. Sepin
203 North LaSalle Street
#1320
Chicago, IL 60601
312/541-1550

**American Dental Hygienists'
Association**
Executive Director: Mr. Stanley B. Peck
444 North Michigan Avenue
Suite 3400
Chicago, IL 60611
312/440-8900

American Dental Interfraternity
Executive Secretary: Dr. Charles D. Fuszner
2800 College Avenue
Suite 286
Alton, IL 62002
618/474-7201

**American Dental Society of
Anesthesiology**
Executive Secretary: Mr. R. Knight Charlton
211 East Chicago Avenue
Suite 810
Chicago, IL 60611
312/664-8270

American Endodontic Society, Inc.
Executive Director: Dr. Ramon Werts
1440 North Harbor Boulevard, Suite 719
Fullerton, CA 92635
714/870-5590

American Equilibration Society
Executive Director: Mr. Sheldon Marcus
8726 North Ferris Avenue
Morton Grove, IL 60053
847/965-2888

American Institute of Oral Biology
Executive Director: Dr. Daryl Ward
620 Glenneyre Street
Laguna Beach, CA 92651
714/497-1250

American Prosthodontic Society
Executive Director: Dr. Alan C. Keyes
919 North Michigan Avenue
Suite 2460
Chicago, IL 60611
312/944-7618

American Society for Geriatric Dentistry
Executive Director: Dr. Aldo D. Boccia
211 East Chicago Avenue
Suite 948
Chicago, IL 60611
312/440-2660

**American Society for the Advancement
of Anesthesia in Dentistry**
Executive Director: Dr. David Crystal
PO Box 551
Bound Brook, NJ 08805
732/469-9050

**American Society for the Study of
Orthodontics**
Executive Director: Ms. Daisy Buchalter
5012 Clearview Expressway
Flushing, NY 11364-1041
718/224-8898

**American Society of Dentist
Anesthesiologists**
President: Dr. John Yagiela
Loma Linda University
School of Dentistry
1092 Anderson, Room 4411
Loma Linda, CA 92350
909/558-4611

**American Society of Dentistry for
Children**
Executive Director: Dr. Peter J. Fos
875 North Michigan Avenue
Suite 4040
Chicago, IL 60611
312/943-1244

**American Society of Forensic
Odontology**
President: Dr. Susan Rivera
11 Tiffany Place
Saratoga Springs, NY 12866-9706
518/584-2342

American Society of Retired Dentists
Executive Director: Ms. Edna Boulanger
1 West Camino Real Boulevard
Suite 207
Boca Raton, FL 33498
561/395-2773

American Student Dental Association
Executive Director: Ms. Karen S. Cervenka,
  CAE
211 East Chicago Avenue
Suite 1160
Chicago, IL 60611
312/440-2848

Association of State and Territorial Dental Directors
Executive Director: Mr. Clay D. Tyeryar
1015 15th Street
Suite 403
Washington, DC 20005-2605
202/408-1254

Christian Dental Society
Secretary: Dr. Mike Roberts
PO Box 296
Sumner, IA 50674
800/237-7368

College of Diplomats to the American Board of Orthodontics
Executive Director: Ms. Elizabeth Matterson
427 Kenwood Avenue
Delmar, NY 12054
518/439-0981

Delta Dental Plans Association
President/CEO: Ms. Kim E. Volk
1515 West 22nd Street
Suite 1200
Oak Brook, IL 60521
630/574-6001

Delta Sigma Delta Fraternity
Executive Director: Dr. John Prey
West 323 South 3380 Hwy F
Dousman, WI 53118
414/968-2030

Dental Assisting National Board, Inc.
Executive Director: Ms. Cynthia C. Durley
676 North St. Clair
Chicago, IL 60611
312/642-8507

Dental Dealers of America, Inc.
Executive Director: Dr. Edward B. Shills
123 South Broad Street
Suite 2030
Philadelphia, PA 19109-1020
215/731-9975

Diving Dentists Society
Executive Director: Dr. Don-Neil Brotman
8105 McDonogh Road
Pikesville, MD 21208
410/363-0530

Federation of Special Care Organizations
Executive Director: Dr. Robert O. Henry
211 East Chicago Avenue
Suite 948
Chicago, IL 60611
312/440-2660

Flying Dentists Association
Executive Director: Ms. Winnie Houston
PO Box 189
Buena Park, CA 90621
714/994-1212

Hispanic Dental Association
Executive Director: Ms. Sandy Reed
188 West Randolph Street
Suite 1811
Chicago, IL 60601
312/577-4013

Indian Dental Association (USA)
Executive Director: Dr. Chandurpal Genhani
3540 82nd Street
Flushing, NY 11372
718/639-0192

National Alliance for Oral Health
Coordinator: Ms. Margot Maganias Thomas
State University of New York at Buffalo
School of Dentistry
355 Squire Hall
Buffalo, NY 14214
716/829-3556

For More Information

National Association of Seventh-Day Adventist Dentists
Executive Director: Dr. Judson Klooster
PO Box 101
Loma Linda, CA 92354
909/824-4633

National Association of Dental Laboratories
Executive Director: Mr. Terry Peters, CAE
8201 Greensboro Drive
Suite 300
McLean, VA 22102
703/610-9035

National Association of Filipino Dentists of America
Executive Director: Dr. Manuel M. Cunanen
3411 West Shore Road
Warwick, RI 02886
401/737-7715

National Dental Association
Executive Director: Mr. Robert Johns
3517 16th Street NW
Washington, DC 20010
202/588-1697

National Dental Hygienists Association
President: Kimberly L. Boyd
7821 South Calumet Avenue
Chicago, IL 60619
773/488-3692

National Foundation of Dentistry for the Handicapped
Executive Director: Dr. Larry Coffee
1800 Glenarm Place
Suite 500
Denver, CO 80202
303/534-5360

Omicron Kappa Upsilon
Executive Director: Dr. Jon B. Suzuki
7703 Floyd Curl Drive
San Antonio, TX 78284
210/567-3160

Organization of Teachers of Oral Diagnosis
President: Dr. Leann Truesdale
PO Box 100412
University of Florida
Gainesville, FL 32610
352/392-1299

Pierre Fauchard Academy
Secretary/Treasurer: Dr. Richard A. Kozal
PO Box 803330
Las Vegas, NV 89188
702/365-9454

Psi Omega Fraternity
Executive Director: Dr. James A. Rivers
1040 Savannah Highway
Charleston, SC 29407
803/556-0573

Sigma Epsilon Delta Dental Fraternity
Executive Director: Ms. Nathan Massoff
Box 278
Great Neck, NY 11022
516/482-0679

Sigma Phi Alpha Dental Hygiene Honor Society
President: Ms. Brenda Parton
University of San Antonio
Department of Dental Hygiene
7703 Floyd Curl Drive
San Antonio, TX 78284
210/567-8820

Sleep Disorders Dental Society
Executive Director: Ms. Mary Beth Rogers
11676 Perry Highway
Suite 1204
Wexford, PA 15090
724/935-0836

Society for Occlusal Studies
President: Dr. Bernard T. Williams
1010 Carondelet Drive
Kansas City, MO 64114
816/941-7330

Society of American Indian Dentists
President: Dr. George Blue-Spruce Jr.
PO Box 15107
Phoenix, AZ 85060
602/231-0078

Xi Psi Phi Fraternity
Executive Director: Dr. Keith Winfield Dickey
1623 Washington Avenue
Suite 300
Alton, IL 62002
618/463-1889

Trade Associations
American Dental Trade Association
President & CEO: Mr. Nikolaj M. Petrovic, CAE
4222 King Street West
Alexandria, VA 22302
703/379-7755

Dental Manufacturers of America
Executive Director: Dr. Edward B. Shils
123 South Broad Street
Suite 2030
Philadelphia, PA 19109
215/731-9975

DENTAL SCHOOLS
The schools in your geographic area may provide information about practitioners or any other dental subject. You may also seek treatment from the schools.

Active Dental Schools (by State)
The following addresses are maintained by the ADA Council on Dental Education, 211 East Chicago Avenue, Chicago, IL 60611, 312/440-2698. Information on graduate programs can be obtained from the same department, 312/440-2669.

Alabama
University of Alabama
School of Dentistry
1919 Seventh Avenue, S.
Birmingham, AL 35294
Dean: Dr. Mary Lynne Capilouto
205/934-4720

California
University of the Pacific
School of Dentistry
2155 Webster Street
San Francisco, CA 94115
Dean: Dr. Arthur A. Dugoni
415/929-6400

University of California, San Francisco
School of Dentistry
513 Parnassus Avenue, S-630
San Francisco, CA 94143-0430
Dean: Dr. Charles Bertolami
415/476-1323

University of California, Los Angeles
School of Dentistry
10833 Lecone Avenue, Room 53-038
CHS
Los Angeles, CA 90095-1668
Dean: Dr. No-Hee Park
310/825-7354

University of Southern California
School of Dentistry
University Park—MC 0641
Los Angeles, CA 90089-0641
Dean: Dr. Harold Slavkin
213/740-2800

Loma Linda University
School of Dentistry
Loma Linda, CA 92350
Dean: Dr. Charles J. Goodacre
909/824-4683

Colorado
University of Colorado Medical Center
School of Dentistry
4200 East Ninth Avenue, Box C-284
Denver, CO 80262
Dean: Dr. Howard M. Landesman
303/315-8752

Connecticut
University of Connecticut
School of Dental Medicine
263 Farmington Avenue
Farmington, CT 06032
Dean: Dr. Peter J. Robinson
860/679-2808

District of Columbia
Howard University
College of Dentistry
600 W Street, NW
Washington, DC 20059
Dean: Dr. Charles F. Sanders
202/806-0019

Florida
University of Florida
College of Dentistry
PO Box 100405
Gainesville, FL 32610-0405
Dean: Dr. Frank A. Catalanotto
352/392-2946

Nova Southeastern University
College of Dental Medicine
3200 South University Drive
Fort Lauderdale, FL 33328
Dean: Dr. Seymour Oliet
954/262-1612

Georgia
Medical College of Georgia
School of Dentistry
1459 Laney Walker Boulevard
Augusta, GA 30912
Dean: Dr. David R. Myers
706/721-0211

Illinois
Northwestern University Dental School
240 East Huron Street
Chicago, IL 60611-2972
Dean: Dr. Lee M. Jameson
312/503-6837

Southern Illinois University
School of Dental Medicine
2800 College Avenue
Building 273/Room 2300
Alton, IL 62002
Dean: Dr. Patrick Ferillo
618/474-7120

University of Illinois at Chicago
College of Dentistry
801 South Paulina Street
Chicago, IL 60612
Dean: Dr. Bruce S. Graham
312/996-1040

Indiana
Indiana University
School of Dentistry
1121 West Michigan Street
Indianapolis, IN 46202-5186
Dean: Dr. Lawrence I. Goldblatt
317/274-7957

Iowa
University of Iowa
College of Dentistry
Dental Building
Iowa City, IA 52242
Dean: Dr. David C. Johnsen
319/335-7144

Kentucky
University of Kentucky
College of Dentistry
800 Rose Street—Medical Center
Lexington, KY 40536-0084
Dean: Dr. Leon A. Assael
606/233-5786

University of Louisville
School of Dentistry
Health Sciences Center
Louisville, KY 40202
Dean: Dr. John Williams
502/852-5293

Louisiana
Louisiana State University
School of Dentistry
1100 Florida Avenue, Building 101
New Orleans, LA 70119
Dean: Dr. Eric J. Hovland
504/619-9961

Maryland
University of Maryland
Baltimore College of Dental Surgery
Dental School
666 West Baltimore Street, Room 4-A-11
Baltimore, MD 21201
Dean: Dr. Richard R. Ranney
410/706-7460

Massachusetts
Harvard School of Dental Medicine
188 Longwood Avenue
Boston, MA 02115
Dean: Dr. R. Bruce Donoff
617/432-1401

Boston University
Henry M. Goldman School of Graduate
   Dentistry
100 East Newton Street
Boston, MA 02118
Dean: Dr. Spencer N. Frankl
617/638-4700

Tufts University
School of Dental Medicine
One Kneeland Street
Boston, MA 02111
Dean: Dr. Lonnie H. Norris
617/636-7000

Michigan
University of Detroit Mercy
School of Dentistry
8200 West Outer Drive, Box 98
Detroit, MI 48219-0900
Interim Dean: Dr. H. Robert Steinman
313/494-6621

University of Michigan
School of Dentistry
1234 Dental Building
Ann Arbor, MI 48109-1078
Dean: Dr. William E. Kotowicz
313/763-6933

Minnesota
University of Minnesota
School of Dentistry
515 SE Delaware Street
Minneapolis, MN 55455
Dean: Dr. Peter Polverini
612/625-9982

Mississippi
University of Mississippi
School of Dentistry—Medical Center
2500 North State Street
Jackson, MS 39216-4505
Dean: Dr. J. Perry McGinnis
601/984-6000

Missouri
University of Missouri—Kansas City
School of Dentistry
650 East 25th Street
Kansas City, MO 64108
Dean: Dr. Michael J. Reed
816/235-2100

Nebraska
Creighton University
School of Dentistry
2500 California Street
Omaha, NE 68178
Dean: Dr. Wayne W. Barkmeier
402/280-5060

University of Nebraska Medical Center
College of Dentistry
40th & Holdrege Streets
Lincoln, NE 68583-0740
Dean: Dr. John Reinhardt
402/472-1344

New Jersey
University of Medicine and Dentistry of New
   Jersey
New Jersey Dental School
110 Bergen Street
Newark, NJ 07103-2425
Acting Dean: Dr. Cecile Feldman
973/972-4300

New York
Columbia University
School of Dental and Oral Surgery
630 West 168th Street
New York, NY 10032
Dean: Dr. Allan J. Formicola
212/305-2500

New York University
College of Dentistry
345 East 24th Street
New York, NY 10010-4099
Dean: Dr. Michael C. Alfano
212/998-9800

State University of New York at Buffalo
School of Dental Medicine
325 Squire Hall
Buffalo, NY 14214
Dean: Dr. Louis J. Goldberg
716/829-2821

State University of New York at Stony Brook
School of Dental Medicine
Rockland Hall
Stony Brook, NY 11794-8700
Interim Dean: Dr. Russell J. Nisengard
516/632-8950

For More Information

North Carolina
University of North Carolina at Chapel Hill
School of Dentistry
104 Brauer Hall, 211 H
Chapel Hill, NC 27599-7450
Dean: Dr. John W. Stamm
919/966-1161

Ohio
Ohio State University
College of Dentistry
305 West 12th Avenue
Columbus, OH 43210
Dean: Dr. Henry W. Fields, Jr.
614/292-9755

Case Western Reserve University
School of Dentistry
2123 Abington Road
Cleveland, OH 44106
Dean: Dr. Jerold S. Goldberg
216/368-3200

Oklahoma
University of Oklahoma
College of Dentistry
PO Box 26901
Oklahoma City, OK 73190
Dean: Dr. Steven K. Young
405/271-6326

Oregon
Oregon Health Sciences University
School of Dentistry–Sam Jackson Park
611 SW Campus Drive
Portland, OR 97201
Dean: Dr. Sharon P. Turner
503/494-8801

Pennsylvania
Temple University
School of Dentistry
3223 North Broad Street
Philadelphia, PA 19140
Dean: Dr. Martin F. Tansy
215/707-2803

University of Pennsylvania
School of Dental Medicine
4001 West Spruce Street
Philadelphia, PA 19104
Dean: Dr. Raymond Fonseca
215/898-8961

University of Pittsburgh
School of Dental Medicine
3501 Terrace Street
Pittsburgh, PA 15261
Acting Dean: Dr. Thomas Braun
412/648-8760

Puerto Rico
University of Puerto Rico
School of Dentistry
Medical Sciences Campus
PO Box 365067
San Juan, PR 00936-5067
Dean: Dr. Fernando Haddock
787/758-2525

South Carolina
Medical University of South Carolina
College of Dental Medicine
171 Ashley Avenue
Charleston, SC 29425
Dean: Dr. Richard W. DeChamplain
803/792-3811

Tennessee
Meharry Medical College
School of Dentistry
1005 D.B. Todd Boulevard
Nashville, TN 37208
Acting Dean: Dr. John Maupin, Jr.
615/327-6489

University of Tennessee
College of Dentistry
875 Union Avenue
Memphis, TN 38163
Dean: Dr. William F. Slagle
901/448-6200

Texas
Baylor College of Dentistry
Texas A&M University Systems
3302 Gaston Avenue
Dallas, TX 75246
Dean: Dr. James Cole
214/828-8201

University of Texas
Health Science Center at Houston
Dental Branch
6516 John Freeman Avenue
Houston, TX 77030
Dean: Dr. Ronald Johnson
713/500-4021

University of Texas
Health Science Center at San Antonio
Dental School
7703 Floyd Curl Drive
San Antonio, TX 78284-7914
Dean: Dr. Kenneth L. Kalkwarf
210/567-3160

Virginia
Virginia Commonwealth University
VCU School of Dentistry
PO Box 980566
Richmond, VA 23298-0566
Dean: Dr. Ronald J. Hunt
804/828-3784

Washington
University of Washington–Health Sciences
School of Dentistry
Room D-322, Box 356365
Seattle, WA 98195
Dean: Dr. Paul B. Robertson
206/543-5982

West Virginia
West Virginia University
School of Dentistry
The Medical Center, PO Box 9400
Morgantown, WV 26506-9400
Dean: Dr. James Koelbl
304/293-2521/22/23

Wisconsin
Marquette University
School of Dentistry
PO Box 1881
Milwaukee, WI 53201
Dean: Dr. William K. Lobb
414/288-6500

Canadian Programs (by Province)
Alberta
University of Alberta
Department of Oral Health Sciences
Room 3036 Dentistry-Pharmacy Building
Edmonton, Alberta T6G-2N8 Canada
Associate Dean: Dr. G. Wayne Raborn
403/492-3117

British Columbia
University of British Columbia
Faculty of Dentistry
350-2194 Health Science Mall
Vancouver, British Columbia V6T-1Z3 Canada
Dean: Dr. Edwin H.K. Yen
604/822-5323

Manitoba
University of Manitoba
Faculty of Dentistry
780 Bannatyne Avenue
Winnipeg, Manitoba R3E-OW3 Canada
Dean: Dr. Johann de Vries
204/789-3631

Nova Scotia
Dalhousie University
Faculty of Dentistry
5981 University Avenue
Halifax, Nova Scotia B3H-3J5 Canada
Dean: Dr. William MacInnis
902/494-2274

Ontario
University of Toronto
Faculty of Dentistry
124 Edward Street
Toronto, Ontario M5G-1G6 Canada
Dean: Dr. B.J. Sessle
416/979-4301

University of Western Ontario
Faculty of Medicine and Dentistry
1151 Richmond Street
London, Ontario N6A-5C1 Canada
Acting Dean: Dr. S.L. Kogon
519/661-3330

Quebec

Ecole de Medecine Dentaire
Université Laval
Pavillon de Medecine
Ste-Foy, Quebec G1K-7P4 Canada
Dean: Mme. Diane Lachapella
418/656-5303

McGill University
Faculty of Dentistry
3460 University Street
Montreal, Quebec H3A-2B2 Canada
Dean: Dr. James Lund
514/398-7227

Université de Montreal
School of Dental Medicine
C.P. 6128 Succursale A
Montreal, Quebec H3C-3J7 Canada
Dean: Dr. Jean Turgeon
514/343-6005

Saskatchewan

University of Saskatchewan
College of Dentistry
107 Wiggins Road, Room B526
Saskatoon, Saskatchewan S7N-5E5 Canada
Dean: Dr. Charles G. Baker
306/966-5119

AMERICAN DENTAL ASSOCIATION GEOGRAPHIC CONSTITUENT SOCIETIES

You may want to ask specific leaders or other individuals in these organizations any questions you have about dentistry.

American Dental Association Constituent Societies

The following addresses are maintained by the Department of Dental Society Services, 211 East Chicago Avenue, Chicago, IL 60611, 312/440-2598. Contact the individual societies below for more information about their meetings.

Alabama Dental Association

Executive Director: Mr. Wayne McMahan
836 Washington Street
Montgomery, AL 36104
334/265-1684

Alaska Dental Society

Executive Director: Ms. Martha Reinbold
9170 Jewel Lake Road
Suite 203
Anchorage, AK 99502
907/563-3003

Arizona State Dental Association

Executive Director: Mr. Greg McFarland
4131 North 36th Street
Phoenix, AZ 85018
602/957-4777

Arkansas State Dental Association

Executive Director: Mr. Billy W. Tarpley
2501 Crestwood Road
Suite 205
North Little Rock, AR 72116
501/771-7650

California Dental Association

Executive Director: Mr. Timothy F. Comstock
1201 K Street
14th Floor
Sacramento, CA 95814
916/443-0505

Colorado Dental Association

Executive Director: Mr. Gary J. Cummins
3690 South Yosemite Street
#100
Denver, CO 80237
303/740-6900

Connecticut State Dental Association

Executive Director: Mr. Noel Bishop
62 Russ Street
Hartford, CT 06106
860/278-5550

Delaware State Dental Society

Executive Director: Ms. Margaret Novak
200 Continental Drive
Suite 111
Newark, DE 19713
302/368-7634

District of Columbia Dental Society

Executive Director: Mr. C. Jay Brown
502 C Street, NE
Washington, DC 20002
202/547-7613

Florida Dental Association
Executive Director: Mr. Daniel J. Buker
1111 East Tennessee Street, #102
Tallahassee, FL 32308-6913
850/681-3629

Georgia Dental Association
Executive Director: Ms. Martha S. Phillips
Lake Ridge 400, Building 17
7000 Peachtree–Dunwoody Road NE
Atlanta, GA 30328
404/636-7553

Hawaii Dental Association
Executive Director: Mr. Loren Liebling
1345 South Beretania Street
Suite 301
Honolulu, HI 96814
808/593-7956

Idaho State Dental Association
Executive Director: Mr. A. Jerry Davis
1220 West Hays Street
Boise, ID 83702
208/343-7543

Illinois State Dental Society
Executive Director: Mr. Robert A. Rechner
1010 South 2nd Street
Springfield, IL 62704
217/525-1406

Indiana Dental Association
Executive Director: Mr. Douglas M. Bush
PO Box 2467
Indianapolis, IN 46206
317/634-2610

Iowa Dental Association
Executive Director: Mr. Robert W. Harpster
505 5th Avenue, #333
Des Moines, IA 50309
515/282-7250

Kansas Dental Association
Executive Director: Mr. Kevin J. Robertson,
    CAE
5200 SW Huntoon Street
Topeka, KS 66604
785/272-7360

Kentucky Dental Association
Executive Director: Mr. Michael Porter
1940 Princeton Drive
Louisville, KY 40205
502/459-5373

Louisiana Dental Association
Executive Director: Mr. Ward Blackwell
7833 Office Park Boulevard
Baton Rouge, LA 70809
225/926-1986

Maine Dental Association
Executive Director: Ms. Frances C. Miliano
PO Box 215
Manchester, ME 04351
207/622-7900

Maryland State Dental Association
Executive Director: Ms. Elza Harrison, CAE
6450 Dobbin Road
Suite F
Columbia, MD 21045
410/964-2880

Massachusetts Dental Society
Executive Director: Dr. James B. Bramson
2 Willow Street
Suite 200
South Borough, MA 01745
508/480-9797

Michigan Dental Association
Executive Director: Ms. Gerri Cherney, CAE
230 North Washington Square, #208
Lansing, MI 48933
517/372-9070

Minnesota Dental Association
Executive Director: Mr. Richard Diercks
2236 Marshall Avenue
St. Paul, MN 55104
612/646-7454

Mississippi Dental Association
Executive Director: Ms. Connie Lane
2630 Ridgewood Road
Jackson, MS 39216
601/982-0442

Missouri Dental Association
Executive Director: Dr. Jacob J. Lippert
230 West McCarty Street
Jefferson City, MO 65102
573/634-3436

Montana Dental Association
Executive Director: Ms. Mary K. McCue
PO Box 1154
Helena, MT 59624
406/443-2061

Nebraska Dental Association
Executive Director: Mr. Tom Bassett, CAE
3120 O Street
Lincoln, NE 68510
402/476-1704

Nevada Dental Association
Executive Director: Mr. Maurice Astley, CAE
6889 West Charleston, #B
Las Vegas, NV 89117
702/255-4211

New Hampshire Dental Society
Executive Director: Mr. Henry Dougherty
PO Box 2229
Concord, NH 03302
603/225-5961

New Jersey Dental Association
Executive Director: Mr. Arthur Meisel
One Dental Plaza
PO Box 6020
North Brunswick, NJ 08902
732/821-9400

New Mexico Dental Association
Executive Director: Mr. Rick Murray
3736 Eubank Boulevard NE
Suite C1
Albuquerque, NM 87111-3556
505/294-1368

Dental Society of the State of New York
Executive Director: Mr. Roy Lasky
4th Floor, 121 State Street
Albany, NY 12207-1622
518/465-0044

North Carolina Dental Society
Executive Director: Ms. Faye Marley
PO Box 4099
Cary, NC 27519
919/677-1396

North Dakota Dental Association
Executive Director: Mr. Joseph J. Cichy
PO Box 1332
Bismarck, ND 58502
701/223-8870

Ohio Dental Association
Executive Director: Ms. Nancy Quinn, CAE
1370 Dublin Road
Columbus, OH 43215
614/486-2700

Oklahoma Dental Association
Executive Director: Mr. Bob D. Berry, CAE
629 West Interstate 44, Service Road
Oklahoma City, OK 73118
405/848-8873

Oregon Dental Association
Executive Director: Mr. William Zepp, CAE
17898 SW McEwan Avenue
Portland, OR 97224
503/620-3230

Pennsylvania Dental Association
Executive Director: Mrs. Camille
    Kostelac-Cherry
PO Box 3341
Harrisburg, PA 17105
717/234-5941

**Colegio de Cirujanos Dentistas
de Puerto Rico**
Executive Director: Ms. Myrna Cruz Garay
Avenue Domenech, #200
Hato Rey, PR 00918
787/764-1969

Rhode Island Dental Association
Executive Director: Ms. Valerie G. Donnelly
200 Centerville Road
Warwick, RI 02886
401/732-6833

South Carolina Dental Association
Executive Director: Mr. Hal Zorn
120 Stonemark Lane
Columbia, SC 29210
803/750-2277

South Dakota Dental Association
Executive Director: Mr. Paul Knecht
711 East Wells Avenue
Pierre, SD 57501
605/224-9133

Tennessee Dental Association
Executive Director: Mr. David S. Horvat
2104 Sunset Place
Nashville, TN 37212
615/383-8962

Texas Dental Association
Executive Director: Ms. Mary K. Linn
1946 South 1H35
Suite 400
Austin, TX 78764
512/443-3675

Utah Dental Association
Executive Director: Mr. Monte D. Thompson
1151 East 3900 South, #B-160
Salt Lake City, UT 84124
801/261-5315

Vermont State Dental Society
Executive Director: Mr. Peter Taylor
100 Dorset Street
Suite 18
South Burlington, VT 05403
802/864-0115

Virgin Islands Dental Association
Executive Director: Dr. Henry E. Karlin
PO Box 10422
St. Thomas, VI 00801
340/775-9110

Virginia Dental Association
Executive Director: Dr. Terry D. Dickerson,
   CAE
PO Box 6906
Richmond, VA 23230
804/358-4927

Washington State Dental Association
Executive Director: Mr. Stephen A. Hardymon
2033 6th Avenue, #333
Seattle, WA 98121
206/448-1914

West Virginia Dental Association
Executive Director: Mr. Richard D. Stevens
2003 Quarrier Street
Charleston, WV 25311
304/344-5246

Wisconsin Dental Association
Executive Director: Mr. Dennis J. McGuire,
   CAE
111 East Wisconsin Avenue
Suite 1300
Milwaukee, WI 53202
414/276-4520

Wyoming Dental Association
Executive Director: Mr. Marvin Cronberg
502 South 4th Street
Laramie, WY 82070
307/755-4009

Dental Associations in Canada
Canadian Dental Association
Executive Director: Mr. Jaraine Neilson
1815 Alta Vista Drive
Ottawa, Ontario K1G 3Y6 Canada
613/523-1770

Index

Page numbers followed by f indicate
figures.